YOUR
PSILOCYBIN
MUSHROOM
COMPANION

An **Informative, Easy-to-Use** Guide to
Understanding **Magic Mushrooms:**
From Tips and Trips to Microdosing and
Psychedelic Therapy

————— **Michelle Janikian** —————

Published by:
Ulysses Press
P.O. Box 3440
Berkeley, CA 94703
www.ulyssespress.com

ISBN: 978-1-61243-947-1
Library of Congress Catalog Number: 2019905627

Printed in the United States by Sheridan Books Minnesota
10 9 8 7 6 5

Acquisitions editor: Casie Vogel
Project editor: Claire Sielaff
Managing editor: Claire Chun
Editor: Scott Calamar
Proofreader: Renee Rutledge
Front cover design: Justin Shirley
Back cover photo: Martin Clarke
Interior design and layout: what!design @ whatweb.com
Interior art: mushroom © Alexander_P/shutterstock.com

CONTENTS

PREFACE

The first time I took mushrooms I had no idea what I was getting myself into. I was only 17 but an enthusiastic cannabis consumer, and I thought of mushrooms as a more intense version of that experience. Years later I've learned that many people have that misconception the first time they take magic mushrooms, but it doesn't make it any less of a shock to the system when you start tripping. The "shrooms" I bought and ate in a country club parking lot in northern New Jersey took a long time to kick in. So long, I had been lamenting in my friend's bed that they didn't work on me, and I was bound to this boring earthly world forever.

When the walls of my best friend's bedroom started breathing, I knew it was time to go home. The next thing I did was incredibly stupid, and if you don't read any more of this book, I hope you just learn from the mistake I'm about to reveal. I hugged my friend goodbye in his driveway—wild-eyed—got in my car, and drove home. Even though the drive is only a couple of miles of quiet country road that doesn't permit more than 30 miles per hour, I'm still surprised to this day that I survived.

I made it home before my midnight curfew and spent the rest of the night tripping in my childhood bedroom. Even though I ended up having a powerful experience, I was completely unprepared for the magnitude of magic mushrooms. What I really needed was a book like this to read first, to help me understand the journey I was about to embark on, to prepare for the wide range of experiences and emotions mushrooms can elicit, and most of all, to learn respect for psilocybin and never ever get behind the wheel when they're in my system.

I can't rewrite my own history, but if I can use it to help others take mushrooms safely, then maybe there is a reason I didn't die by crashing into a tree or deer that night. Magic mushrooms have incredible power, and people are inherently curious to try them. They can help you see the world, yourself, and other people in a new light, one that's more accepting, forgiving, or clear. They can cause visions when you close your eyes, and the world around you can seem so much more alive and significant. But they can also be dangerous if special care and preparation aren't taken, and they can be nightmarish if your mind-set and environment—a concept we'll get into known as "set and setting"—aren't taken into consideration.

We're currently in the midst of a psychedelic renaissance, and more people than ever before are curious about trying psilocybin mushrooms and other psychedelics. However, the first wave of psychedelic research and its ensuing enthusiasm got out of control, and we're still recovering from the damage of the 1960s, of widespread psychedelic use without proper preparation. The stigma surrounding psychedelics created back then is still strong today, so how can we be sure not to repeat the mistakes of that era? For starters, we can use psychedelics safely and prepare for the experience by considering the tips in this book and others like it.

More than 12 years after my first mushroom trip and a few years since I touched them at all, I went to a psilocybin mushroom retreat and tripped for healing for the first time. In the course of a week, I was to take mushrooms three times in shamanic ceremony accompanied by group therapy, integration meetings, and yoga and meditation classes. After my first ceremony on 1.5 grams of Golden Teachers, I was ready to give up. Even though I had done a ton of research and wasn't psychedelic-naïve, I had a tremendously challenging experience; I felt completely inadequate and unqualified to write this book, a feeling that had been causing me a constant low-level anxiety for the previous couple months.

I cried for almost the entire trip. It didn't feel like the cathartic experience I'd read about in books and online. Instead of less ego, I got more, and a mean, hateful one at that. I felt totally defeated, and I begged the mushrooms, my subconscious, anyone for answers. Why did I feel this way? Why was I so anxious and disconnected? Why was I so depressed and insecure? I wanted to dig into my past and find the one traumatic event that made me the way I was so everything in my life could be explained and I could move on. Instead, I cried and cried, and the only answer I got was: *"Why" is the wrong question.*

The next day I began to learn the true value of "integration"—a concept I had written about and yet didn't fully understand until I was raw from a challenging psychedelic experience, the first bad trip of my life. For me, integration—processing and learning from my psychedelic experience (see Chapter 11)—began during an unassuming conversation over lunch. But talking about how I felt the night before while someone held space for me changed my outlook incredibly as I moved forward.

I stopped thinking of myself as a reporter there to document the magic mushrooms, let my guard down, and tried to embrace the experience. That's when I really started learning about psilocybin rather than fearing its mysterious power. I also opened myself up to the 17 other retreat participants and stopped seeking so much alone time. At my own pace, I became more comfortable and stopped constantly comparing myself to everyone.

My second ceremony was much more forgiving. I settled back into my yoga mat and pillows and began to go inward—which I was admittedly resisting slightly—and felt tranquil albeit still sad. I thought of my mother and her cancer, my *medzmama* (Armenian for grandmother) and her dementia, and I cried, yet nowhere near as many tears as two days before. But I also realized everything is a choice, and I can choose to be closer to them rather than prematurely grieving their loss. I saw that everything in my life is ultimately my decision, and with this new perspective, I can choose to act differently.

It was a powerful experience, and an incredibly healing one. The next day in our integration meeting I was finally able to share without being choked up by tears. It felt so good, and I was starting to get some of that catharsis that I was looking for and had read so much about. This sense of self-forgiveness extended into the next few days, making it easier to connect and share with people while I wasn't on mushrooms. I felt more comfortable in my own skin, more confident speaking up for myself and asking for things—something that my social anxiety prevented in the past.

This set me up to have an incredible experience during the third and final ceremony, where I took the highest dose of mushrooms of my life: 4 grams. I was determined to go deeper, to stay in my spot with my eyes closed and go inward rather than resist and look at trees or go play with my new friends.

The trip I had is hard to put into words, even though I'm convinced I had a spiritual or mystical experience. I never completely lost my ego, although it felt different. All of my fear and sadness were gone, and I was a ball of light, the laughing Buddha, a goddess who could do anything. I laughed often, and from a deep place in my belly that I didn't even know existed. When I thought of all my doubt surrounding this book, I snorted with laughter and realized "doubt is stupid." I felt like I had everything figured out, from my book to human existence, everything made perfect sense and was hilarious—hilariously obvious.

I remembered that psychedelics could help put people in touch with their "authentic selves," the pure unadulterated person they were born as before life fucked them up and defense mechanisms, like anxiety, got in the way. When I thought of this and the way I was feeling, like a ball of confident light that could do anything if I just stopped being afraid and tried, I felt an incredible relief that the mushrooms chose to show me such a wide range of experiences over the course of a week.

I had been so stressed that I was unqualified to write this book, that I didn't understand mushrooms at all so how could I possibly help others to understand and use them safely? But after that third ceremony I stopped beating myself up. No one knows exactly how mushrooms work, and I saw that I don't need to be the first to figure it out to write this guide. It was an incredibly comforting thought that I'm still trying to integrate as the anxiety of finishing this project in time finds its way back to me. But what I do know, from experience and months of research and interviews, is that mushrooms are incredibly powerful. They can be terrifying and they can be blissful; they can help you see things that the ego prevents you from realizing in everyday life, but they can also be dangerous if you don't pay proper attention to certain things, like thorough preparation and integration. Even though I had heard this quote often before tripping on mushrooms three times in one week, I didn't fully understand it until after: "We don't always have the trip we want; instead, we seem to have the trip we need."

So my beautiful mushroom people, as you embark on preparing for a psychedelic psilocybin experience, whether it be your first trip or your first mindful one, just remember to respect these powerful and magical fungi. And if you do, they can help you find an inner strength and respect for the most important person in this world: you.

PART ONE:

WHAT IS PSILOCYBIN AND HOW DOES IT WORK?

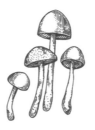

Chapter I

WHAT IS PSILOCYBIN AND WHY USE MUSHROOMS?

WHAT IS PSILOCYBIN?

Nature is filled with extraordinary compounds. Plants produce all kinds of secondary alkaloids, often as a defense mechanism to protect themselves. Yet, scientists are still unsure of the purpose of one of Mother Nature's most mysterious substances: psilocybin. Found in over 180 species of mushrooms in nearly every corner of the globe,[1] psilocybin is a natural psychedelic alkaloid. In the body, it's broken down into psilocin, which causes

---

1   Wikipedia, "List of Psilocybin Mushroom Species."

the psychedelic effects. There is a whole genus of mushrooms that contain psilocybin and psilocin: *Psilocybe*. There are also more psilocybin mushrooms outside of this genera, and some speculate there are even more to be discovered.

The most diverse species of psilocybin-containing mushrooms live in a magical country just south of the US, Mexico. The late Gastón Guzmán, who was a leading expert in *Psilocybes* and the first to discover many psilocybin species, estimated there were 55 different species in Mexico alone. However, his daughter, Laura Guzmán Dávalos, also an esteemed mycologist and professor at the University of Guadalajara in Jalisco, Mexico, tells me there may be even more species in less studied parts of the world, like Central and South America as well as Africa. In fact, she explains that although her father identified over 40 species in the Americas, she believes there are more to be found here, especially in remote, tropical jungles. It's not that far-fetched of an idea considering that many mycologists like Dávalos believe only 3 to 8 percent of the estimated 2.2 to 3.5 million species of fungi have been named and identified at all.

With so many different species of psilocybin mushrooms, are there different magic mushroom experiences? Many psilonauts (those who regularly use magic mushrooms) would argue yes, and indigenous people who use mushrooms ceremonially would probably agree. The indigenous people of the Sierra Mazateca mountain region of Oaxaca, Mexico, believe different mushrooms have their own *fuerza,* or power. "There are certain species that are more prized and coveted," Christopher Casuse, who has been working with the Mazatec for over a decade, tells me. For this reason, different species are employed for different ceremonial uses. Many mushroom users outside of the ceremonial context say something similar, that different types of mushrooms have their own "signature"; some create certain types of visual experiences, physical sensations, or have particularly strong introspective effects, for example.

This variance in experience could be due to the slightly different chemical structures of individual species and strains of shrooms. For instance, different species have varying levels of psilocybin and psilocin. And even among one species, strength varies. *Psilocybe cubensis*, one of the most popular species of psychedelic mushrooms, can have between 0.15 to 1.3 percent psilocybin and 0.11 to 0.5 percent psilocin. And it's considered "moderately potent."[2] Plus, there can be many strains of one species of mushroom, especially among *cubensis*, which are also the most commonly cultivated psilocybin-containing mushrooms. What's more, homegrown varieties can be stronger than naturally occurring strains due to advanced cultivation techniques.

But beyond psilocybin, there are even more secondary alkaloids produced by mushrooms that could be affecting the experience as well, such as baeocystin and norbaeocystin, though more research is needed to say for sure. It could be very similar to the "entourage effect" theory of the cannabis experience. While THC is the dominant alkaloid that produces the cannabis high, many scientists believe it's actually the combined effect of the over 400 compounds found in the plant, including other cannabinoids and flavor-producing terpenes.

However, with psilocybin mushrooms, your environment and mind-set going into the experience may play an even larger role in their effect than the chemical composition of the fungi. A

2   Stamets, *Psilocybin Mushrooms of the World.*

concept known as "set and setting" in the psychedelic community can drastically change the mushroom experience, often referred to as the "trip." We'll explore these ideas in more depth in later chapters, but they're important concepts to get familiar with as we begin this journey.

Speaking of environment, *Psilocybes* grow in a wide variety of settings. While some prefer pastures and cow manure, others thrive on disturbed land in cloud forests. Paul Stamets, a leading authority on psilocybin mushrooms who's identified a few new species, theorizes why they prefer such habitats in his book and identification guide, *Psilocybin Mushrooms of the World*. He writes that, before human civilization, psilocybin mushrooms thrived after ecological disasters like landslides, floods, hurricanes, and volcanoes. "This peculiar affection for disturbed habitats enables them to travel, following streams of debris." Then when humans came into the picture, we were constantly creating ecological disturbances, and so we were the perfect creatures to coevolve with—always creating ideal conditions for shrooms to thrive. Now, psilocybin-containing mushrooms seem to grow at the edge of human civilization, near things like parking lots and graveyards, and they particularly love landscaped areas with mulch, like in front of police stations, causing Stamets to speculate "an innate intelligence on the part of the mushrooms."

Unlike many other secondary alkaloids produced by plants in nature, scientists still don't know exactly what evolutionary advantage the production of psilocybin has for mushrooms. Dávalos explains to me that many alkaloids are produced to prevent animals from eating the plant, so that they can continue to survive. However, with psilocybin, it doesn't seem to be the case, at least not as with other plants, because animals, like deer, still eat psilocybin-containing mushrooms in nature. This has caused many people who have taken them to speculate just the opposite: that psilocybin is produced exactly so animals, especially humans, will consume and experience them. Because of the common trip outcome of returning with a greater appreciation for nature and a stronger urge to protect the planet from contamination, some believe psilocybin is a direct communication link with Mother Nature. And the indigenous people who have used mushrooms ceremonially for centuries believe something similar. Yet, researchers have recently speculated that psilocybin evolved to "mess with insect brains"[3] to protect the mushrooms from attack,[4] because fungi and bugs can compete for the same food, like dung and decaying wood.

Lastly, it's important to note that psilocybin-containing mushrooms aren't the only psychoactive mushrooms that produce a trip. The second most famous is *Amanita muscaria*, also known as the fly agaric, the picturesque, large, red-capped mushroom with white spots. *Amanita muscaria* and other species of the *Amanita* genus produce a different psychoactive compound, muscimol, which results in a very distinct trip compared to psilocybin, and one that's less popular among recreational users. According to Dávalos, one of the main characteristics of its experience is the sensation of being very small while the rest of the world seems huge. It's the reason many cultures associate this mushroom with elves, gnomes, and dwarves, because it can make you feel like one for a while. Like *Psilocybes*, *Amanitas* have also been used ceremonially, for instance, by shamans in ancient Siberian

---

3   Frazer, "Magic Mushroom Drug Evolved."
4   Reynolds, "Horizontal Gene Cluster Transfer."

culture.[5] Dávalos tells me there are even more psychoactive mushrooms in nature, but with no known ceremonial uses.

WHY DO PEOPLE USE MUSHROOMS?

Contrary to popular belief, people of all walks of life use mushrooms occasionally for a variety of reasons; their use isn't limited to hippies and some kind of druggie subculture. I learned this firsthand both interviewing people for this book and attending a psilocybin mushroom retreat where I took the sacred fungi with 17 other people of all age groups and backgrounds, many of whom were previously psychedelic-naïve. But why do 60-year-old grandparents and 29-year-old publicists eat magic mushrooms?

The answers are as individual as the people, but some common themes keep popping up. For one, I continue to hear that mushrooms give people a "reset"; some describe this as an emotional reset, others as a reset on their creativity, but they all use this term that scientists at the Imperial College London have also been exploring in their psilocybin research (more on this in Chapters 3 and 4)[6]. Another popular reason commonly heard in the psychedelic community is eating mushrooms for personal or spiritual growth. This again can mean different things to different people, but the idea is the same: adults using mushrooms with the intention to learn more about themselves and, maybe, become better or happier people. Compared to

---

5   Letcher, *Shroom: A Cultural History.*
6   O'Hare, "Magic Mushrooms May 'Reset.'"

other psychedelics, mushrooms particularly help people see themselves more clearly, or at least from a new angle, and that can help folks make actionable changes in their lives after their trip.

Of course, not everyone is looking to change their lives or their minds with mushrooms. In fact, according to a survey conducted by longtime psychedelic researcher and author of *The Psychedelic Explorer's Guide*, James Fadiman, a large portion of people do mushrooms for fun and out of curiosity. Unlike others in the psychedelic community, I'm not going to say that there's anything wrong with using mushrooms recreationally, as long as you do so safely and mindfully. If you take the proper precautions like the ones outlined in this book, and you don't harm anyone else in the process, I believe it's your right to expand your mind on mushrooms even if the law doesn't agree. While I am in no way encouraging anyone to do anything illegal, I'm also not trying to contribute to the stigma of these fungi or make them exclusive, inaccessible, or overly medicalized.

In fact, a few recent studies have found that lifetime psychedelic use outside of clinical trials is associated with reduced psychological distress and suicidality in American adults in comparison to users of other drugs[7, 8]—whether that use be recreational, ceremonial, or for personal growth is unknown. This is important because a lot of emphasis is put on doing mushrooms in a controlled environment, like a clinical trial, for positive outcomes, but these studies show that people doing psychedelics at home or in ceremony are also benefiting. However, it's important to note, modern psychedelic users, or

7   Hendricks, et al., "Classic Psychedelic Use Is Associated."
8   Johansen and Krebs, "Psychedelics Not Linked to Mental Health."

"psychonauts," are very conscious of ideas like set and setting and have more often than not created their own controlled, safe environments and rituals to ensure safe journeys.

That being said, there's a lot of talk in the media about psilocybin possibly being a solution to a lot of serious mental health issues like depression, anxiety, post-traumatic stress disorder (PTSD), addiction, and obsessive-compulsive disorder (OCD), among others. While this is real research with serious promise, getting these results at home on your own might be less likely, even after creating a safe environment. If you are looking to do mushrooms for healing, I would highly recommend seeking out professionals to help you do so successfully. There are a few options, like attending retreats abroad, finding an underground therapist, or applying to participate in clinical trials, and I explain each in more depth in Chapter 6.

However, both experts and mushroom enthusiasts attest that mushrooms help us access self-healing or an "inner healing intelligence." Even a few occasional mushroom users I interviewed for this book spoke of this, like Ashley Manta, sex coach and CannaSexual creator, who primarily uses mushrooms to help her access self-love and acceptance. It's a use I'm familiar with personally, because mushrooms can help me turn off my inner critics and find love and appreciation for the person I am when everything is stripped away. This same experience is why some people use mushrooms for positivity, reset, anxiety, and even depression. It can also help people who previously thought they had a lack of direction or motivation to find it within themselves. Yet, a big part of using mushrooms for personal growth is "integration," which we'll get to in Chapter 11, but the key is remembering these insights and the positive, self-love feelings during your everyday life to help give you strength and confidence.

IS PSILOCYBIN SAFE?

For three years running, the Global Drug Survey has found "magic" psilocybin-containing mushrooms to be the safest "illicit" substance.[9] That's because mushrooms put the least amount of people in the hospital when compared to other drugs, even LSD. The survey, which is the largest in the world and annually asks over 100,000 people in over 30 countries about their substance use, has continuously found that less than 1 percent of over 10,000 mushroom users seek emergency medical treatment due to their trips. The survey findings also point out that picking and eating mushrooms in nature is riskier than tripping, because misidentification of a poisonous species is known to harm more people per year than psilocybin itself. What's more, it would be very difficult to overdose on psilocybin, and there have been no recorded fatalities of doing so.

In fact, mushrooms' relative safety has caused some prominent researchers to suggest that the US government reschedule psilocybin from Schedule I to Schedule IV.[10] At the moment, shrooms are a Schedule I substance in the US, meaning they are considered one of the strongest, most addictive drugs that lacks any sort of medical value. But although, physically, psilocybin is very safe, its mental impact may be another story. Tripping can induce anxiety, bring repressed emotions to the

---

9   Global Drug Survey. www.globaldrugsurvey.com
10   Johnson, et al., "The Abuse Potential of Medical Psilocybin."

surface, and cause confusion. So that's how psilocybin can be dangerous: when people become a threat to themselves or others or do thoughtless and risky things while under its influence. However, with proper preparation, special attention paid to a safe supportive environment, and possibly a sitter or guide—all of which we'll discuss in depth later on in this book—mushrooms can be very safe and rewarding. Plus, according to the Drug Policy Alliance,[11] psilocybin is not addictive and does not trigger compulsive use.

The only other thing that makes mushrooms dangerous is their legal status. Even though *Psilocybes* grow naturally on every continent, their possession, use, and cultivation is illegal in most countries, including the United States. Therefore, it's probably more dangerous to be caught with psilocybin mushrooms than it is to ingest them, even though that is beginning to change with recent decriminalization initiatives.

Are magic mushrooms safe? When I ask one of the most prominent and long-standing psychedelic researchers, Bill Richards, who has guided hundreds of journeys, he says it's very much like skiing or swimming. If you don't have some guidance and instruction, you can really hurt yourself, but we don't make skiing illegal. So if you're planning a magic mushroom trip, read this guide carefully and take its advice to heart. If you adequately prepare for your journey, you should avoid any unnecessarily dangerous situations or outcomes. And you could end up with one of the most meaningful experiences of your life.

---

11   Drug Policy Alliance. www.drugpolicy.org/drug-facts/are-psilocybin-mushrooms-addictive

Chapter 2

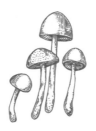

INDIGENOUS CEREMONIAL MUSHROOM USE

There is a world beyond ours, a world that is far away, nearby, and invisible. And there is where God lives, where the dead live, the spirits and the saints, a world where everything has happened and everything is known.

—María Sabina, famous Mazatec curandera

Anthropologists speculate both *Psilocybes* and *Amanitas* have been used ceremonially by cultures for thousands of years.[12] In fact, cave paintings in Algeria's Tassili n'Ajjer national park in the Sahara desert that date back to between 6000 and 4500 BCE are speculated to represent the psychoactive effects of psilocybin

---

12   Samorini, "The Oldest Archaeological Data."

mushrooms and perhaps their ritual, shamanic ingestion.[13] In the Americas, sacred mushroom use is more concrete. Mushroom stones dating as far back as 3000 BCE that have been uncovered in ancient Mayan territories of Guatemala and southern Mexico are thought to represent a pre-Hispanic mushroom cult.[14] However, these ceremonies still exist to this day in current indigenous villages of the Mexican states of Oaxaca, Puebla, and Michoacán.[15]

Deep in the Sierra Madre mountains of Oaxaca, the most famous ceremonial use of magic mushrooms continues with the Mazatec people. So much can be learned about psilocybin's safe and sacred use from the Mazatec rituals, which are hundreds of years old. In their community, a select number of individuals are called to become *curanderos*, or healers, and even fewer still are called to work with the most revered of all holy plants: the sacred mushroom. I spoke with a Mazatec man, Inti García Flores, a local professor who has been working to preserve and archive the sacred traditions of his hometown, Huautla de Jiménez, Oaxaca, since he was six years old. He tells me it's usually later in life that people receive the calling to pursue healing work, often after surviving or being healed from a grave illness themselves. He explains that the path to *curandismo* is a process—it doesn't happen in a year, nor does it happen after eating mushrooms one time. Often, the word of their community's ancient deities, *los chikones*, the "wise guardians of the mountains, rivers, paths, and wells," manifests itself in their dreams, and in time, gives them the word and the power to pursue healing, García Flores says.

---

13   Samorini, "The Oldest Representations of Hallucinogenic Mushrooms."

14   Carod-Artal, "Hallucinogenic Drugs in Pre-Columbian."

15   Schultes, *Plants of the Gods.*

Similarly, it's a long, diagnostic process for a member of the community to receive a sacred mushroom ceremony. In Mazatec culture, mushrooms are used for healing illness, both physical and mental. But in modern times, it is a last resort, both after seeing other curanderos and Western medical professionals. "You don't go directly to the mushrooms," García Flores explains. First, you may go to other wise people in the community, like an oracle to "have your corn read" or to others who "read copal," a local tree resin that is burned ceremonially throughout Mexico and Central America. If these traditions can't help you, then you will be sent to a curandero who specializes in mushrooms.

García Flores gives me another example of the modern diagnostic process, a personal story of his mother's cancerous tumor. Their first call of action was to go into the city to an oncologist, who removed the tumor from his mother. Then the entire family went together to the curandero for a mushroom ceremony, which is the traditional way to see a healer: as a complete family. Together, they prayed and asked the mushrooms, "What was the cause of this tumor? What was the problem? Why did the disease choose their mother?" The ceremony raises the sick family member up, to encourage the individual to solve their problem. That was many years ago, but recently, when they returned to the city for tests, they learned his mother's tumor had not metastasized, even though she had not adhered to any special diet or other types of follow-up treatment, besides, of course, the mushroom ceremony.

When mushrooms are eaten ceremonially, the Mazatec people believe they are communicating directly with the chikones. "The chikones are the protectors of the hills, of the rivers, caves, forests, and mountains that are here in the Sierra Mazateca.

And each *chikon* has their own special function in the ceremony," García Flores tells me. He explains that during the ritual, participants are "opening the hill" and asking the chikones for help, typically healing for themselves or their family members. If you ask from your heart, with sincerity and lots of love, they will listen to you and give you what you want. The chikones are also at the heart of the sacred mushrooms' origins in Mazatec culture. García Flores tells me, "Grandparents, the elderly, have always said the mushrooms are a gift from Naichaun, who is the spirit of thunder. That when it thunders is when the mushrooms sprout here, when they are born it is a gift from Naichaun."

But what is the actual ceremony—known as a *velada* or *desvelada* in Spanish—like? While each curandero has their own style, certain rituals are obeyed. For instance, ceremonies are only held at night, and there are some days that are better for healing than others. García Flores tells me Tuesdays, Thursdays, and Saturdays are good days to eat mushrooms, but there are even specific days for different purposes. For instance, some days are better for healing, and others are better for speaking with the dead, another indigenous use of the sacred fungi.

One more standard tradition is the presence of an altar in the ceremony space, which is typically in the curandero's home. Consisting of many candles (*velas* in Spanish), items of significance, and often crosses and other Christian or spiritual symbols, altars are considered a link between the physical and spiritual worlds, and so every item is an expression of that individual's faith. But it was surprising for me to see so much Christian imagery on a magic mushroom curandera's altar in *Little Saints*, a documentary which depicts a psilocybin ceremony in Huautla.[16] In the film, 88-year-old curandera named Natalie performs a velada for a handful of Westerners. Her altar is packed with crosses, dolls of saints, paintings of the Virgen de Guadalupe, and other Christian imagery that is common around Mexico. This is because, since the Spanish colonization of Mexico, many indigenous groups practice a fusion of Catholicism and their more ancient beliefs, known in anthropology as syncretism,[17] and the Mazatec are no exception. Interestingly, while the curanderos believe god speaks to them through the mushrooms, the chikones only speak to indigenous people. "A curandera told me that when a foreigner comes for a ceremony, they only speak with the Western gods. Nothing more. For them, the chikones won't speak," explains García Flores. That makes sense considering the *Little Saints* documentary, in which all of the ceremonial participants were foreigners, so it's not a surprise that the curandera invoked the Christian saints and prayers.

While the standard practice for clinical trials using psilocybin for therapy has some similarities to indigenous ceremony,[18] there are a few interesting differences between Western and indigenous psychedelic healing. For one, rather than have participants close their eyes and "go inward" like in the Western model, in Mazatec culture, participants are encouraged to keep their eyes open and focus on the altar. I ask Christopher Casuse, who works with the Mazatec and who was the one who introduced me to García Flores, about this. Casuse explains that the curandera he's worked with extensively (Natalie from the *Little Saints* documentary) discourages "closing eyes and sinking

16 Quintanilla, *Little Saints: Eat a Mushroom*.

17 Markman and Markman, *Masks of the Spirit*.

18 Johnson, Richards, Griffith, "Human Hallucinogen Research: Guidelines."

back," a process they refer to as "falling out." By keeping your eyes open and focused on the altar she is really trying to train your attention, Casuse says. "You're learning how to work with people while taking the mushroom at the same time. And in order to do that, you need to develop a certain level of vigilance and attention."

The altar and its offerings also play a vital role in this process. "It's a really theoretical tradition that uses sacred images as a gateway for healing," Casuse tells me over the phone. "So focusing on the virgin is a particular type of connection to the divine." In terms Westerners can better relate to, the altar also serves as a distraction of sorts for when your trip gets disconcerting or challenging. "When people get lost in their personal biographical issues, it's like a form of disorientation. People become very confused and get trapped in cycles, but the altar is basically a way to reorient attention," explains Casuse. Another main difference between ceremony and psychedelic therapy is that the curandero is there with you on the journey. He or she also eats the sacred mushroom and acts not only as your guide but as your intermediary to the gods.

There is also intense ritual regarding the mushrooms themselves, which grow wildly in the area during rainy season. For one, the Mazatec believe the fungi are easily contaminated by bad energy. Therefore, no one is supposed to handle or even look at them until it is time for the ceremony. To prevent contamination, the mushrooms, or *hongos* in Spanish, are wrapped in large tamale leaves until they are served.

Many years ago, there was even further ritual involved in keeping the mushrooms pure, García Flores tells me. While they're still picked in the wild and eaten fresh, who actually gathers them has recently changed. In the past, only children were permitted to pick the sacred fungi because they still had an innocence that adults in the community did not. The curandero would go with a child on the full moon to the mountain where the mushrooms grow and say a prayer for permission to cut them. According to the ritual, they would harvest them with great care and affection, singing to the fungi as they wrapped them gently. Then, to further avoid contamination and keep the mushrooms' energy pure, the curandero and child would return to town on lesser-known paths to avoid "bad encounters." Bad encounters would have included seeing a dead animal or a funeral procession on the way. Even seeing a woman, especially a pregnant one, could contaminate the mushrooms, as could seeing a sick person, García Flores says. So the child and curandero would take the road less traveled, so to speak, and then place the wrapped mushrooms carefully on the altar awaiting ceremony. To this day you're not supposed to look at the mushrooms until it's time to eat them in ceremony; because contaminated mushrooms don't do their job, they don't teach the same lessons, explains García Flores.

When it is time for the ceremony, the mushrooms are always served fresh and in pairs within a tamale leaf. The pairs represent the male and female energies, and so an even number must be eaten. In fact, García Flores says if an uneven number of fresh mushrooms are consumed, "they don't teach you anything." And so, to the Mazatecs, pairs of *hongitos* are more important than grams of mushrooms when considering dose. How many pairs you are given is at the discretion of the curandero.

Once the ceremony starts, what is it like? While ceremonial singing and healing seem to go hand in hand, especially when you consider the *Icaro,* or healing song, of ayahuasca ceremonies in South America, Casuse, who has participated in both types of indigenous ceremonies, says song is less of an integral part of the sacred mushrooms ritual. Rather, prayer is more prominent for the Mazatecs. García Flores explains that it really depends on the purpose of the ceremony. For instance, healing ceremonies will have different songs and rituals than ceremonies that intend to speak with the dead. "It depends because the mushrooms will tell you," García Flores says. So whether a particular song— or other type of ritual like the burning of sacred tobacco, San Pedro, or the consumption of cacao—is needed will depend on the ceremony's intention as well as what the mushrooms tell the curandero. "No two ceremonies are alike," says García Flores.

Within the Mazatec community, there are also a few ways participants need to prepare themselves leading up to a ceremony. Especially for healing rituals, partakers need to care for themselves beforehand by not drinking alcohol, eating red meat, smoking tobacco, or having sexual relations, García Flores explains. It's also not advisable to go to a wake or to see a dead body before eating the sacred mushrooms because the fungi are very sensitive and could pick up on that energy.

As far as post-ceremony customs, the community has a couple of expectations for participants in order to keep them safe. For one, it's advised to stay home the day after eating mushrooms. Similar to taking a day of rest after a Western mushroom experience, the Mazatec believe it's best not to go out into the street because participants are very perceptive and their spirits are very sensitive, says García Flores.

But a main difference between post-ceremony expectations in the Mazatec community and the Western world is keeping your experience private. Recently in the West, we've put a lot of emphasis on integrating psychedelic experiences for healing, especially by talking about them in support groups, with friends and family, or with trained therapists. But in order to preserve the sacredness of the ceremony, the Mazatecs don't talk much about their trips. García Flores tells me, the things you learn about your true self, your family, and your sickness are too intimate to share; they are secrets the mushrooms have revealed to you that you have to protect. But that doesn't mean the Mazatecs aren't integrating their experiences—they just don't rely on the talk-therapy aspect like Westerners do. Their culture has already integrated mushroom use, to them it is a holy tradition that is treated with the utmost respect and used sparingly for special purposes. They have a framework for understanding these potentially life-changing ceremonies that doesn't exist in mainstream Western society. And so, by sharing our experiences, perhaps we're compensating for a pillar of the Mazatec community that we lack in our day-to-day, as a way to help us understand and fit this powerful experience into the narrative of our lives.

One last comparison I'd like to make between indigenous and Western use of mushrooms is the lack of abuse in the Mazatec community. Although psilocybin mushrooms aren't addictive like other substances, misuse, such as taking them too often or without preparation, definitely happens in the West. So I ask García Flores if he's heard of anyone in the Mazatec community who abuses mushrooms or uses them outside of the ceremonial context for fun, and he responds with a firm no. But he continues to say that foreigners do abuse mushrooms, even foreigners who live in Huautla, his hometown. "I think it's because they lack, or they're ignorant of, the sacred use," he says. Having a mushroom ceremony as a sacred part of the Mazatec culture has taught the community respect for the experience that Westerners may not appreciate. Which makes me wonder: Could incorporating mushrooms into our own culture also diminish their misuse? Regardless, the ritual use of these revered and magical fungi can teach us a lot, not only about their safe application, but respect for their power and holiness.

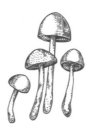

Chapter 3

PSYCHEDELIC THERAPY

A VERY BRIEF HISTORY OF PSILOCYBIN'S ROLE IN PSYCHEDELIC RESEARCH

When psilocybin was first isolated by Swiss chemist Albert Hofmann in 1958,[19] the same scientist who discovered LSD in 1943, psychedelic research was already in full swing. Since the early 1950s, researchers, especially psychologists and psychiatrists, were using LSD and sometimes mescaline to help patients with a variety of conditions. One of the original and

---

19   Carhart-Harris and Goodwin, "The Therapeutic Potential of Psychedelic Drugs."

most well-studied uses of psychedelics was to treat alcoholism,[20] and both private physicians and clinical researchers gave patients psychedelics because, at the time, it was totally legal. In fact, it wasn't until the counterculture's full embrace of the substances that they were stigmatized and then criminalized in 1968. But until that time, there were over 1,000 studies published on LSD's ability to advance psychotherapy that an estimated 40,000 people took part in.[21] Researchers also looked at psychedelics for different types of addictions, "neurosis, schizophrenia, and psychopathy"[22] as well as end-of-life pain and anxiety.[23] Plus, they also gave psychedelics to creatives, scientists, and academics for research and problem-solving.[24] And they even looked at their ability to induce "mystical experiences," like the famous Good Friday Experiment.

Part of the Harvard Psilocybin Project, the Good Friday Experiment was the first study to show psilocybin had the ability to induce "mystical states" after it was given to 10 theology students (and another 10 received niacin, an active placebo) while listening to a two-and-a-half-hour Good Friday mass.[25] Six months later, most of the psilocybin group reported the experience was one of the most spiritually significant of their lives and "increased their involvement with the problems of living and the service of others."[26] When Rick Doblin, founder of the Multidisciplinary Association for Psychedelic Studies (MAPS) followed up with most participants nearly 25 years later,

20 Smart, et al., "A Controlled Study of Lysergide."

21 Richards, *Sacred Knowledge: Psychedelics and Religious Experiences.*

22 Costandi, "A Brief History of Psychedelic Psychiatry."

23 Johnson and Hendricks, "Classic Psychedelics: An Integrative Review"

24 Fadiman, *The Psychedelic Explorer's Guide.*

25 Pahnke, "Drugs and Mysticism."

26 Clarke, W. H. and Funkhouser, G.R. "Physicians and Researchers Disagree."

all of those who received psilocybin continued to characterize the experience as "one of the high points of their spiritual life."[27]

Although indigenous communities have been experiencing this mystical state during mushroom ceremonies for thousands of years, the Good Friday Experiment was the first to highlight the importance of mystical experiences in a clinical context. Bill Richards, who was a close friend of the experiment's author, Walter Pahnke, tells me, "In the context of science, it was the first study to really demonstrate that psilocybin does something unique. That it's not just expectation and suggestion and responding to beautiful music." And now, these ineffable, spiritual experiences are believed to play a big part in how psychedelics work to elicit change and healing.

WHAT IS PSYCHEDELIC THERAPY?

Psychedelic therapy was developed in the 1950s as one of two treatment modalities using psychedelic substances. The other is called psycholytic therapy, and the difference really comes down to dose. In psychedelic therapy, a large dose of a psychedelic is given, equivalent to around 5 to 7 grams of dried psilocybin mushrooms, in order to induce a mystical experience that is seen as a catalyst to change, according to Richards's book *Sacred Knowledge*. In psycholytic therapy, much smaller doses are given (typically 20 to 70 micrograms of LSD, which is similar to 0.5 to 2 grams of dried mushrooms depending on the fungi's strength)

---

27   Doblin, "Pahnke's 'Good Friday Experiment.'"

in order to open up the patient more during talk therapy and access feelings and memories that are harder to discuss when sober.[28] In both treatment modalities, the patient is always under the compassionate supervision of a therapist or two during the drug session or sessions, and in the weeks preceding and following, in order to establish rapport as well as to continue to unpack or "integrate" the psychedelic experience.

Today, the use of psychedelics in clinical trials looks a lot more like the psychedelic therapy modality where one or more high-dose drug sessions are given with the intention of eliciting a spiritual experience. In fact, scientists are even finding that the more "mystical" a person's trip is, the more effective the therapy.[29] We'll get into that more in the next chapter on how psilocybin works, but any researcher will tell you that the preparation and controlled safe setting of clinical psychedelic therapy plays a large role in its efficacy as well.

I spoke with Peter Hendricks, psychologist, professor, and psychedelic researcher at the University of Alabama at Birmingham, who is currently conducting a study on psilocybin for cocaine addiction, to see exactly what psychedelic therapy looks like in clinical trials. Hendricks says, first, potential participants are screened for disqualifying medical conditions like hypertension or a history of "severe persistent mental illness." Once selected, participants in his cocaine-dependency study have four separate two-hour-long therapy sessions to build rapport with their two co-therapists, who will eventually facilitate their dosing session. Having two therapists present, typically one

---

28   Hofmann, *LSD, My Problem Child.*

29   Johnson and Hendricks, "Classic Psychedelics: An Integrative Review."

male and one female, is a staple of psychedelic therapy that you don't see very often in regular talk therapy.

During these rapport-building sessions, therapists ask participants leading questions to get to know them better, things like: Where did you grow up? What's your relationship like with your mother? "For every person we see, there is a complex universe and experience behind their eyes, and we want to know what that is," says Hendricks. The point is not only to get to know the person and their experience, but to really make sure they feel understood, heard, and cared for. He explains this is because when participants are under the influence of psilocybin, it's crucial that they feel safe and "completely at ease" so they can feel comfortable enough to "trust, let go, and be open to completely surrendering themselves to that experience." If participants feel unsafe or uncared for in any way on drug-administration day, they are much more likely to resist psilocybin's effects and therefore have a challenging trip without the transformative effect that comes from relinquishing control. In this particular study, participants are also provided with cognitive behavioral therapy (CBT) in order to "give them some skills to better cope with the urge to use cocaine," says Hendricks.

Then, there is one high-dose drug-administration session in Hendricks's trial. In other recent studies, this part of the therapy can differ. For instance, the team at Imperial College London often gives participants one low to medium dose first, then one high dose a week or so later.[30] And Matthew Johnson at Johns Hopkins has also recently tweaked this part of the therapy in his smoking-cessation trial to include one moderate dose, one high

---

30 Carhart-Harris, et al., "Psilocybin with Psychological Support for Treatment-Resistant Depression."

dose, and then the option to receive a third high dose only if the participant wants.[31]

The drug-administration session is typically done indoors in a pleasant room decorated to look like a cozy living room with some spiritual highlights like a statue of the Buddha. There's always a big, comfortable couch where participants are encouraged to lie down and wear an eye mask and headphones that play music chosen by the researchers. And that's how most of the six-to-eight-hour dosing session looks. Participants can get up and walk around, go to the bathroom, or have a drink of water, but they're actually encouraged not to do much talking while they're under the influence—that comes later. Therapists will check in with the participant occasionally, and hold their hand if it looks like they're struggling, but they are also encouraged not to talk much, but rather to be a calm and supportive presence that encourages the participant to "go inward."

The first "integration," or debriefing session, comes the next day, but Hendricks tells me many participants begin talking about their experiences at the end of the dosing session. Then, the following day, they really begin to unpack the trip and talk about any lessons or realizations they came to during the experience. "Often they know that there's meaning and very often they can see what that meaning is immediately," says Hendricks. "Other times it takes them time to unpack the experience, think about the narrative in depth and begin to understand what it means to them." He explains that their lessons are often much more than stopping cocaine use: "It's about being the best versions of themselves that they can be… A lot of it also applies to eating well and exercising, and being a better father, mother, brother,

31 Johnson, "Long-Term Follow-Up."

grandparent." Then, there are four more two-hour sessions where participants continue to unpack the trip, work on CBT skills, and plan any next steps they need to take to improve themselves.

While all clinical trials using psilocybin—to my knowledge—have a debriefing session the day following the drug experience, not all trials have the same amount of integration sessions. The debriefing also allows researchers to check participants for any adverse reactions to the psilocybin, like lasting visual distortions, which, knock on wood, Hendricks says they haven't seen so far. The amount of integration sessions differs from trial to trial because it really depends on what the psilocybin is being used to treat. But also because, as Hendricks points out, "the science is emerging. There are so many questions we don't have the answer to." In the future, the treatment will probably be more standardized, especially if it's legally available. But for now, scientists are trying to figure out what works best for people, and there are a lot of exciting trials on the horizon.

THE PSYCHEDELIC RENAISSANCE: CURRENT AND FUTURE STUDIES

Many have been referring to the current resurgence of psychedelic research as the "psychedelic renaissance." After psychedelics were made a Schedule I substance in 1970, most research into their benefits was halted and any therapeutic use was pushed underground. Bill Richards was one of the last psychologists to continue psychedelic research at the Spring

Grove State Hospital in Baltimore, but even they were shut down in 1976.[32] It wasn't until the 1990s that clinical investigations slowly started up again, first in Rick Strassman's lab with DMT, the psychedelic compound in ayahuasca.[33]

The first clinical trial using psilocybin in the US since the '70s came in 2006, when researchers at Johns Hopkins University published a groundbreaking paper in the *Journal of Psychopharmacology*: "Psilocybin can occasion mystical-type experiences having substantial and sustained personal meaning and spiritual significance."[34] Not to oversimplify things, but this paper, with its meticulous study design and fascinating results, jump-started modern psychedelic research as we know it. Essentially a modern version of Pahnke's Good Friday Experiment, not only did no one get hurt after receiving a high dose of psilocybin (in the psychedelic therapy conditions mentioned above), but 67 percent considered the experience one of the top five most significant of their lives, and 61 percent of participants met the criteria for having a complete mystical experience.

When the Johns Hopkins team followed up with participants a year later and asked them to fill out a standard personality test,[35] they made a significant discovery: Most criteria remained the same, except in the category of "openness." What they found was those who had mystical experiences were now statistically more open,[36] which is meaningful for two reasons. The first being

---

32   Yensen and Dryer, "Thirty Years of Psychedelic Research."

33   Strassman and Qualls, "Dose-Response Study of N,N-dimethyltryptamine."

34   Griffiths, et al., "Psilocybin Can Occasion Mystical-Type Experiences."

35   Costa and McCrae, "Revised NEO Personality Inventory."

36   MacLean, Johnson, and Griffiths, "Mystical Experiences Occasioned by the Hallucinogen."

that the average person's personality doesn't evolve much past age 30, and so finding a substance-induced experience that could change people is radical. Second, all of the traits associated with openness, like "sensitivity, imagination and broad-minded tolerance of others' viewpoints and values," are powerfully positive and predicative of an emotionally mature and well-functioning person.

Since that study, many more have followed, at Johns Hopkins and at other well-respected universities around the country and the entire world. Later in 2006, scientists looked at the safety and efficacy of psilocybin for obsessive-compulsive disorder (OCD),[37] and their results were promising. That same year, another group of researchers reviewed a set of curious data, self-reports on the successful use of psilocybin and LSD to treat cluster headaches, which are famously painful and hard to get rid of.[38] Unlike the majority of psychedelic research in the 1950s and '60s which was done with LSD, now psilocybin had taken main stage. Michael Pollan reports that was because the word "psilocybin" carried less political baggage than "LSD."[39] Even at the time of writing this book, the only recent studies looking at LSD are outside of the US.

The next landmark study to come out was in 2011 for the use of psilocybin for end-of-life anxiety, another application they began to investigate in the mid-twentieth century.[40] At UCLA, psychiatrist Charles Grob and his team gave 12 terminally ill cancer patients who also had clinical anxiety due to their

---

37   Moreno, et al., "Safety, Tolerability, and Efficacy."

38   Sewell, Halpern, and Pope, "Response of Cluster Headache to Psilocybin and LSD."

39   Pollan, *How to Change Your Mind.*

40   Costandi, "A Brief History of Psychedelic Psychiatry."

diagnosis a "moderate" dose of psilocybin. Their findings were also positive, with a significant reduction in anxiety for over three months and increase in mood for over six.[41] This study has since been replicated with positive results at NYU[42] and Johns Hopkins,[43] and it's been cause for many in the psychedelic community to question the way we die in Western society. If psilocybin becomes rescheduled in the future, members of the community have proposed building centers where those with terminal illness could go to use psychedelics legally, possibly even with their loved ones.[44] That's because a main theme for many of the participants in these trials is realizing how important their relationships are, how their response to their illness is negatively affecting the people they love, and that they want to spend the last chapter of their lives enjoying the presence of others.[45] "It helps people live until they die," Richards tells me, "not just lie in their beds, feeling sorry for themselves and preoccupied with pain. It could transform palliative and hospice care dramatically in the next few years. It's a very exciting frontier."

Recently, there have also been studies looking at psilocybin for addiction and smoking cessation, with more planned for the future, especially looking at psilocybin for opioid dependence.[46] There has also been a lot of recent research into how psilocybin works in the brain using advanced imagining techniques that didn't exist during the first wave of psychedelic

---

41   Grob, et al., "Pilot Study of Psilocybin Treatment."

42   Ross, et al., "Rapid and Sustained Symptom Reduction."

43   Griffiths, et al., "Psilocybin Produces Substantial and Sustained Decreases."

44   MacLean, "Open Wide and Say Awe."

45   Dauber, *A New Understanding: The Science of Psilocybin.*

46   Heffter Reseach Institute. heffter.org/future-research

research.[47] Interestingly, the researchers spearheading these neuropsychological studies at Imperial College London have also found that people with treatment-resistant depression are greatly benefiting from psilocybin sessions,[48] and that's expected to be a major avenue of research considering how many people worldwide are affected.

While most pharmaceutical companies have stayed hands-off because psilocybin occurs in nature and so therefore is not patentable,[49] there are some nonprofit organizations as well as for-profit companies currently funding this research. The Usona Institute is one, and they're currently recruiting participants for a large-scale upcoming phase II clinical trial testing psilocybin for treatment-resistant depression,[50] part of the FDA's four-step drug approval process. If all phases are successfully completed, psilocybin could be on track to become a regulated medicine in the US.

The other main organization funding research in the US is the Heffter Research Institute, and their website lists a lot of interesting projects they'd like to support, including psilocybin for:

- anorexia
- Alzheimer's disease
- stress-induced depression and anxiety
- post-traumatic stress disorder (PTSD)

47 Imperial College London. www.imperial.ac.uk/people/r.carhart-harris/publications.html

48 Carhart-Harris, "Psilocybin for Treatment-Resistant Depression."

49 Farah, "Inside the Push to Legalize."

50 Usona Institute. https://usonaclinicaltrials.org/major-depressive-disorder-psilocybin-clinical-trial-psil201

- MDMA vs. psilocybin therapeutics: study evaluating the similarities and differences between MDMA and psilocybin therapies
- emotion, creativity, and cognition: research on psilocybin enhancing creativity and cognition
- psilocybin group therapy process: examination of psilocybin group therapy process and outcomes
- spiritual vs. non-spiritual: study of psilocybin effects in "spiritually-oriented" vs. "non-spirituality-oriented" volunteers
- psilocybin vs. mushrooms: comparison of chemically synthesized psilocybin with psilocybin naturally occurring in mushrooms
- SSRI (selective serotonin reuptake inhibitor)-psilocybin interaction: study on how psilocybin interacts with SSRI antidepressants

The possibilities for psilocybin research are seemingly infinite, yet scientists at the moment are being extremely cautious. Back in the '60s, it was the researchers themselves who took psychedelics out of the clinical context and into the counterculture, like Timothy Leary. Now, scholars are excited and hopeful, but careful to curb their enthusiasm; they don't want to encourage people to try this stuff at home and cause another cultural backlash.

However, it's exciting nonetheless. "I could spend the rest of my life, my career trying to answer some of these questions, as can those who come after me, and there are still many decades of research on psilocybin that will follow," says Hendricks. When I ask him at the end of our hour-long phone conversation if there's any future studies he'd like to see, he says, "Oh boy that list is endless." However, he does tell me he'd like to see some work with psychedelics for chronic pain like fibromyalgia. "But thinking outside the box, in many ways, the applications could be limitless."

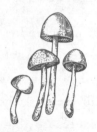

Chapter 4

HOW PSILOCYBIN WORKS

Everything about psilocybin is mysterious, especially how it works. How does it create that mystical trippy feeling? How does it change people? How does it work in the brain? And how are these reactions connected? These are complicated questions with many answers, and all of them are just theories at the moment. In this chapter we'll explore the different subjective experiences psilocybin can produce and how they motivate people toward personal growth. We'll also explore the current theories on what's happening in the brain and why that might possibly create both the acute trip and lasting change that it does. We'll also touch on mystical experiences, the most ineffable and arguably most valuable of the possible trip outcomes.

First of all, it's important to recognize that we don't exactly know what's happening when people take psilocybin. But with the psychedelic renaissance has also come interest in trying to answer some of these big questions—not only how psychedelics work, but how consciousness works at all.

While there are finally scientific studies looking at brain scans of people while they're tripping on psychedelics to try and create a better understanding of how they function, the individual's subjective experience still seems to hold the most weight for personal growth. That's because these experiences are often filled with insight, lessons, and new perspectives. When I ask Peter Hendricks about this, about why something as "unscientific as a mystical experience" seems to help people the most, he compares psychedelic experiences to antidepressants. "If you give someone an SSRI, they may not notice much of anything," Hendricks says. "Very subtly over a period of time they say, 'Oh yeah, I guess I do feel better.' And we can say, 'Oh yeah, that's because we've tinkered with your serotonin levels in your brain.' But from people who had experiences with psychedelics, they'd say, 'My God, that was profound and salient. And I can tell you why I think I changed... from my perspective, it's because I had this experience. It was very memorable and meaningful and motivated me to change my behavior or allowed me to see things from a new perspective that has since had very beneficial impacts on my life.'" Put another way, in the words of Ros Watts from a study she sent me, "During psilocybin, people often accessed new perspective and revelations that helped them *turn insights and understandings into actions* [sic]."[51]

These insights and revelations can come for people at different doses and intensities of experiences, but one of the most interesting aspects of psychedelic research is that participants in

51   Watts and Luoma, "The Use of the Psychological Flexibility."

clinical trials seem to benefit the most from psychedelic therapy when they have full-on "mystical, spiritual, or peak" experiences during dosing sessions. When I speak with Richards about this phenomenon, he first points out that other types of psychedelic experiences are still valuable and therapeutic. Especially at low and medium doses, people have what Richards calls a "psychodynamic or psychological experience" where they deal with things like grief, guilt, anger, interpersonal relationships, and conflicts, as well as experiences of age regression and confrontations of life trauma that can all be incredibly healing and helpful.

This is often what is referred to as things "bubbling up" during a psychedelic experience that need to be dealt with. While on higher doses people can experience transcending these old wounds, that's not always the case, especially at low and medium doses. However, you don't need to transcend these feelings for them to be beneficial. Sometimes, it's enough to just recognize—from a new perspective—that these are things in your life that are bothering you, and you can take that knowledge back with you to work on.

But at higher doses, and when people feel comfortable and trusting enough in their set and setting to completely let go and embrace the experience, that's when another type of healing can occur that's often described as a mystical or peak experience. But what is a mystical experience? Richards has defined "mystical consciousness" in his book, *Sacred Knowledge*, and in his many talks on the subject. But basically it includes six qualities:

1. Unity: a sense of oneness with all things

2. Transcendence of time and space: as if these earthly concepts are irrelevant

3. Intuitive knowledge: a sense of being privy to the secrets of the universe that you've known all along

4. Sacredness: a profound sense of homecoming and a natural connection to the divine

5. Deeply felt positive mood: "euphoria" doesn't even begin to describe it

6. Ineffability: impossible to put the experience into words, often because it's so paradoxical

Richards has also distinguished between two types of mystical experiences, and this is where the notion of "ego dissolution" comes into play. Basically, there are two levels to these psychedelic-fueled spiritual experiences: one where you're still you, or your ego is still intact, and then a higher level where you lose yourself completely and often, contentedly. While both experiences are usually accompanied by feeling a deep connection to all things, during the ego-loss peak experience, people report losing their sense of "I" and becoming one with humanity, nature, the entire universe, god, love, or nothingness.

But what's most curious in clinical trials with psilocybin is that participants who have the most mystical experiences, as defined by the Mystical Experience Questionnaire (MEQ), a peer reviewed psychological scale,[52] also seem to benefit the most from

---

52   MacLean, "Factor Analysis of the Mystical."

psychedelic therapy, no matter if the study is for addiction[53] or end-of-life anxiety.[54] But why?

"Clearly it's more than just momentarily feeling good, not just getting high," Richards tells me over Skype. He explains that the memory of these transcendental experiences can change people by changing their concept of the self. "After that experience, you know that you are more than this being that walks through the world, pays bills, and eats three meals a day. That there really is a mystery within us," Richards says. "You can label it different ways. But there is a sense of connection, that there is something deep within us that's incredibly beautiful, trustworthy, and more real or fundamental than this state of consciousness." He outlined this idea during a presentation in 2017,[55] that the memory of a mystical experience is helpful for the following reasons:

1. Change in self-concept

2. Enhanced self-worth

3. Fresh awareness of "inner resources"

4. Sense of personal empowerment

5. Enhanced perception

Watts also describes this "shift in self-concept." Participants in her trial describe being "able to bypass their ordinary conceptualized self, with its daily concerns, and contact other, newer perspectives, including an observer self, teacher self, wise self, and a loving compassionate self... This expanded sense of

---

53 Garcia-Romeu, Griffiths, and Johnson, "Psilocybin-Occasioned Mystical Experiences."

54 Ross, S., et al., "Rapid and Sustained Symptom Reduction."

55 Richards, "Sacred Knowledge: Just Because."

self brought a new sense of confidence, assurance, and a sense of being looked after, loved, and feeling more consistently supported."[56] Richards tells me a similar idea: "One of the insights, besides—if you will—the reality of 'the secret,' is there is beauty and worth within you. So it makes it very hard to maintain low self-worth, or to pretend that you're not valued, you're not important."

This same notion, that there is something powerful, knowledgeable, and beautiful within us, is often called our "inner healing wisdom" or "intelligence" by the psychedelic community. Sometimes, this can take the form of an "inner vision quest" when you're actually under the influence of psilocybin, where you can confront challenging aspects of yourself, like your "shadow" (a concept we'll explore more in Chapter 10), or your past, especially traumatic events. This inner healing wisdom can also take the form of insights and realizations as well as physical manifestations, like shakes, pain, or nausea. "That's one of the most amazing things to me about this whole field," Richards says, "how the mind of just about everyone—not just those with a doctorate in English literature—how the human mind choreographs experiences for the individual person that what emerges is intrinsically well structured and meaningful to teach you something." Richards explains that this idea comes back to the teachings of the prominent early-twentieth-century psychologist Carl Jung. Jung worked with dreams and the mental imagery that arose during deep relaxation states and found a meaningful process would unfold. With psychedelics, it's that same principle, says Richards.

---

56   Watts, et al., "The Use of the Psychological Flexibility."

Another way researchers have tried to explain how psychedelic experiences—especially mystical ones—work for personal growth is through the sensation of awe. Hendricks explains it to me in a way that was very similar to Richards's idea of change in self-concept. Basically, during strong psychedelic experiences, "our attention is so acutely focused on something that is unlike anything we've ever experienced that there's almost a sort of liberation from our self-nagging thoughts. So if we're talking about end-of-life anxiety and you're ruminating in an almost pessimistic way about your future, then having an experience in which all of your attention is directed toward something else for a period of time, you might feel like you've been released from this sort of ruminative rut...You might return feeling like, wow, you're just not that worried about it anymore," Hendricks says. This is similar to the idea of an emotional reset that many people who use psilocybin talk about, and that Watts and the Imperial College London team have found participants to experience as a sort of "defragging" of their brains.[57] But Watts warns me over the phone that she doesn't know if it's healthy for people to go into a psilocybin experience expecting their brains to be biologically reset, because that's not exactly how it works. She emphasizes the analogy of a clinically controlled psychedelic experience being like 10 years of therapy in one day, because it's more about the insights and realizations, the new perspective you have access to, and how you're going to use that to change your everyday life.

Hendricks echoes this sentiment, that the component of insight psychedelic experiences can provide is crucial to how they work. "Imagine someone who's been addicted to cocaine for a period

---

57   Watts, et al., "Patients' Accounts of Increased 'Connectedness.'"

of time," he tells me. "They have this profound realization [during a psilocybin session] that, 'my God, I have burned so many bridges. I've alienated so many people. I've affected and damaged so many relationships all for this drug. What the heck am I doing? I need to change my ways because you know, life is not about me and what I want, but it's about our connections with others.'" It's a common insight that people come to on psychedelics; that human connection and love are the keys to a fulfilled and happy life. Hendricks compares it to the realization that Ebenezer Scrooge has during Charles Dickens's famous novella, *A Christmas Carol*. After his perspective-shifting experiences with the three ghosts who visit him on Christmas Eve, Scrooge sees he's focused all of his time and energy on money, and in doing so, ruined relationships and hurt other people along the way. He realizes he doesn't want to leave that legacy, and Hendricks says, after "peak" psychedelic experiences, many people feel the same. "There's an insight or introspection or reorientation toward the world wherein your own concerns take a back seat to the concerns of others."

This is very similar to a finding that Watts and her team found at Imperial College London: that part of how psychedelic experiences work to change people is through an increased sense of connectedness. During their trial on psilocybin for treatment-resistant depression, they noticed a similar theme among participants, that after psilocybin-assisted therapy they felt more connected to themselves, others, and the world in general.[58] The study's authors point out that a common feature among many psychiatric disorders is a sense of disconnection or isolation, especially depression and addiction. Yet, their

58   Carhart-Harris, et al., "Psychedelics and Connectedness."

participants reported feeling "reconnected to past values, pleasures, and hobbies as well as feeling more integrated, embodied, and at peace with themselves and their often troubled backgrounds. It is a working hypothesis of ours that connection-to-self is a bedrock form which connection to others and the world can follow most naturally," Watts and her colleague Robin Carhart-Harris, head of the Centre for Psychedelic Research at Imperial College London, write. They continue to emphasize this connection to the self as helping people access a wider range of emotions, or reconnecting depressed people with their feelings by moving from "emotional avoidance to acceptance."

Does this feeling of increased connection originate in the peak experience of being at one with the universe? Considering the feeling of homecoming that many have during psychedelic mystical experiences, it certainly seems related. As Richards explains it: "There's a sense of belonging [during a unitive experience], so you can't feel totally estranged and isolated anymore. Like, good news! You belong to the human family!" Yet, Watts adds that this sense of increased connection in depressed participants might come more from the intensity of the therapy portion of their psychedelic therapy protocol. Participants in their trial at Imperial College London were depressed for an average of 18 years before receiving psilocybin-assisted therapy. In the past, these people only received the standard mental health care services in the UK, which generally consists of six therapy sessions and, often, a prescription to antidepressants, like SSRIs. But with psychedelic therapy, she explains, it's a very long and intense process where therapists and clients form deep connections. And so, perhaps their feelings of reconnection are more a result of the interpersonal relationships they formed with the two therapists and "having been a part of something that was really significant to them," says Watts. It's an interesting question to ponder, but one can't help but draw a connection to what we're learning about what happens in the brain when you take psilocybin.

THE BRAIN ON PSILOCYBIN

Advancements in the past few years have revolutionized our understanding of how psilocybin works in the brain. The prevailing theory also comes from Imperial College London's Psychedelic Research Centre where in 2012, Carhart-Harris and colleagues began scanning the brains of study participants on psilocybin using fMRI, expecting to find an increased amount of activity. What they found instead was a substantial decrease in activity in brain regions that make up the Default Mode Network (DMN). In fact, the more intense the trip, the less activity they saw in the DMN.[59] But what does this mean? What does the DMN even do in "normal" waking life?

The DMN, sometimes referred to as the gravity center of the brain,[60] is responsible for the high-level aspects of consciousness that essentially make us human, like sense of self, worry,[61] self-referential thinking, autobiographical memory, conceiving the perspective of others, planning for the future,[62] moral decision-

---

59   Carhart-Harris, et al., "Neural Correlates of the Psychedelic State."
60   Davey and Harrison, "The Brain's Center of Gravity."
61   Watts, et al., "Patients' Accounts of Increased 'Connectedness.'"
62   Buckner, et al., "The Brain's Default Network."

making,[63] and self-consciousness.[64] The DMN helps us tell the story of ourselves, or our "ego," as well as navigate social situations by using past experiences to help us make decisions and plan for the future. "It helps you to identify and codify what is important to you, what you value, what you fear, what you dislike," says James Giordano, professor of neurology and biochemistry at Georgetown University Medical Center. The DMN is a big part of what distinguishes us from other mammals, but an overactive system is also thought to be responsible for things like excessive rumination and overly negative self-critical thoughts that are common in mental health conditions like depression, anxiety, addiction, obsessive-compulsive disorder, eating disorders, and others.

And so what happens when you turn the volume down on your Default Mode Network? While on psilocybin, instead of staying stuck in the same old narrative—or having the same parts of the brain communicate—now the brain makes new, novel connections (see Figure 1), a theory Carhart-Harris has dubbed the "entropic" or "anarchic" brain theory.[65] This action is where researchers believe most of the acute subjective effects, like ego dissolution and insights, as well as visual and auditory distortions, lie, not to mention the root of psilocybin's potential for personal growth. That's because, researchers like Watts and Carhart-Harris speculate, it is in this psilocybin-induced "chaotic" state that the brain becomes more flexible and less dominated by the everyday narrative we tell ourselves, which, in the case of some psychiatric conditions, are actually harming us and holding us back. In recent years, Carhart-Harris has refined

63   Kaplan, et al., "Processing Narratives Concerning Protected Values."
64   Fingelkurts, et al., "DMN Operational Synchrony Relates."
65   Carhart-Harris, et al., "The Entropic Brain."

this theory, now calling it the REBUS model (Relaxed Beliefs Under pSychedelics)[66]— theorizing that when psychedelics relax our DMN and its "high-level beliefs," then the brain has more communication with older, instinctual parts of itself, like the limbic system. "This liberated upwards limbic flow can disrupt unhelpful entrenched beliefs," writes Watts.[67] "Instead of being constrained to a small number of 'gravitationally dominant attractors', the mind and brain freely transitions between states, which can feel like the mind is 'opening up.'"

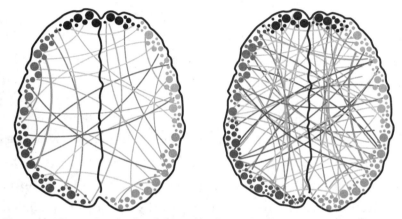

Normal brain communication (left) and brain communication on psilocybin (right). Image is a re-creation of Imperial College of London's findings.

In this same article, Watts explains this theory in terms of an analogy of a snowplow evening out snow on a ski slope. "Our brain is like a skier that ordinarily follows the well-trodden tracks," Watts writes. "The psilocybin experience can temporarily disrupt and flatten the old grooves in the snow, setting up the possibility that new tracks may be laid down. Essentially psychedelic administration can foster new, short-term flexibility and the ability to start new habits of thinking, acting, and

66   Carhart-Harris and Friston, "REBUS and the Anarchic Brain."

67   Watts and Luoma, "The Use of the Psychological Flexibility."

feeling." She goes on to explain that these new habits must be practiced in order to "consolidate new learning," basically explaining the importance of integration (which we'll get to in Chapter 11). "In other words," Watts writes, "the new tracks need to be worn well enough to prevent one from reverting to old tracks too easily." Basically, your ingrained day-to-day narrative of yourself is disrupted, giving you the opportunity to see yourself and your world differently for the duration of the trip. It makes sense, considering how people describe psychedelics as giving them a "new perspective" or a "new self-concept," to use Richards's language, but what you do with that new perspective depends on your actions moving forward. And so, even if your brain is altered for a few hours, it's up to you to take these insights and apply them to your life in order to enact any personal growth. Simply taking mushrooms alone likely won't change who you are, but if you practice new ways of being, maybe you won't get stuck in the same rut.

But how do mushrooms quiet the Default Mode Network? It all has to do with the brain's serotonin system. Let's back up a little. When you eat magic mushrooms or take a psilocybin capsule, it's actually metabolized into the prodrug psilocin. When psilocin reaches your brain, it triggers the serotonin system, specifically the serotonin receptor: 5-HT2A (which we'll just call the 2A receptor from now on). Unsurprisingly, the brain regions with the most 2A receptors are part of the Default Mode Network,[68] and thus part of our "higher level" brain systems. When psilocin acts on 2A receptors, it initiates the quieting of the DMN and the novel brain connections that follow. Basically 2A receptors

---

68   Beliveau V., et al., "A High-Resolution in Vivo Atlas."

are psychedelics' "trigger point."[69] In fact, researchers have found that if 2A receptors are "turned off" first, like if using a 2A antagonist, then psychedelics don't produce the signature "mind revealing" effect.[70]

Serotonin 2A receptors play a role in a lot of really interesting behaviors. For instance, Carhart-Harris writes that 2A signaling has been shown to play a role in cognitive flexibility.[71] There have also been links between "trait pessimism," like "pathological brooding" and deficient 2A receptor stimulation.[72, 73, 74, 75] Both of these roles of 2A receptors make sense considering how people use psychedelics for personal growth, but some of the most interesting links between the serotonin system and psychedelics have to do with neural plasticity. Essentially, researchers have found evidence that 2A signaling may enhance neural plasticity, meaning that psychedelics may be able to promote brain plasticity by acting on those receptors.

But what is neural plasticity exactly? Basically, it used to be believed that the brain stopped changing structurally after childhood, but now scientists know that the brain continues to change and adapt based on things like learning, environment, and even damage. There are two types of neuroplasticity, Giordano points out: functional plasticity and structural plasticity. Functional plasticity is the brain's ability to redirect functions from a damaged area of the brain to a healthier one.

69   Carhart-Harris and Friston, "REBUS and the Anarchic Brain."

70   Vollenweider, et al., "Psilocybin Induces Schizophrenia-Like Psychosis."

71   Boulougouris, et al., "Dissociable Effects of Selective 5-HT$_{2A}$."

72   Carhart-Harris, et al., "Neural Correlates of the Psychedelic State."

73   Bhagwagar, et al., "Increased 5-HT(2A) Receptor Binding."

74   Meyer, et al., "Dysfunctional Attitudes and 5-HT2 Receptors."

75   Farb, et al., "Mood-Linked Responses in Medial."

Structural plasticity, on the other hand, is the brain's capacity to change its physical structure often as a result of learning. And scientists at the University of California, Davis, found that psilocin and other psychedelics are able to promote both kinds of plasticity in cortical neurons.[76]

This is important for a few reasons, but the researchers themselves indicate that a common physical symptom of depression and other related mental health conditions is the atrophy of neurons in the prefrontal cortex, an area of the brain that plays a large role in mood, emotion, and anxiety regulation. What they found was that psychedelics like psilocin, LSD, and DMT were able to robustly promote neuritogenesis (new growth from neurons), therefore potentially counteracting depression's detrimental effect on those same neurons. What's more, they found that this same process is mediated by our favorite serotonin receptors: 2A. And so Carhart-Harris has recently theorized that when the brain enters its "entropic" state on psychedelics where the DMN is quieted, it creates a "window of high plasticity" that may be able to change the brain even once the psychedelic substances have worn off.[77]

So how does psilocybin work? It appears to have a twofold approach. Its effect on the brain not only gives people access to a new perspective, insights, and lessons they can use to better their lives, but sometimes even full-blown mystical experiences that can change their sense of self-concept and motivate them to be the best versions of themselves. That same process also seems to have potentially long-lasting structural effects on our brains, especially those under siege of depression and other similar

76   Calvin, L., et al., "Psychedelics Promote Structural and Functional."
77   Carhart-Harris and Friston, "REBUS and the Anarchic Brain."

conditions. It's not two separate actions but one fully integrated experience, especially if you've prepared a supportive and safe set and setting. It's mystical to say the least, and amazing that this is all from a substance found in fungi that grow wild around the world.

PART TWO:

HOW TO TRIP SAFELY AND EFFECTIVELY

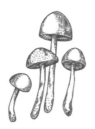

Chapter 5

HOW TO PREPARE YOUR SET AND SETTING

WHAT IS SET AND SETTING?

"Set and setting" is a phrase coined by the most infamous of psychedelic researchers and psychonauts, Timothy Leary, in his 1964 tripping manual *The Psychedelic Experience*, and it has stuck around ever since. "Set" refers to a person's mind-set while "setting" indicates their physical and social environment, both of which drastically affect how a psychedelic trip plays out. That's because, while under the influence of a psychedelic like psilocybin-containing mushrooms, you become very sensitive to both your internal experience and external environment. And so, to avoid an unnecessarily bad or stressful trip, you must plan ahead for optimal set and setting conditions.

HOW TO CHOOSE THE RIGHT SETTING

Choosing the ideal setting for your trip will depend on your intentions, but there are a few things to consider while planning your journey. First of all, it's crucial that your setting is comfortable, safe, and familiar, which is why a lot of people prefer to trip at home, especially for their first time. Your setting will greatly affect your set, and so if your situation is chaotic, loud, distressing, or even messy, it can have an immense impact on your sensitive state of mind. Physically, it's important to have a cozy place to sit and lie down, with bathroom access. Mentally, you need to feel secure in this space so you can confidently release your control to the mushrooms without any underlying anxiety. You also want to make sure there are no strangers coming and going because the presence of other people, tripping or sober, can have a big impact on your trip.

That's why the next thing to decide is whether you want to take mushrooms with other people or by yourself (ideally with a trip sitter). While there are pros and cons to each, deciding which situation is best will really depend on your intentions for the experience. Tripping with friends, loved ones, and significant others can be a profound bonding experience. Especially in small groups or one-on-one, mushrooms can help people connect on incredibly deep and lasting levels. In fact, through my research for this book, I had several people reach out to me explaining that they fell in love with their partner on mushrooms and are still together now, years later. It's also nice to have friends and loved ones to not only go through the journey with, but with whom to talk about it and integrate it after the fact. If you do decide to trip with others, make sure to keep the group size small and to communicate your intentions and expectations beforehand as well as any boundaries or anxieties you might have. Because you're in such a vulnerable state, you really only want to trip with those you are very close with. If it's your first time tripping and you don't want to do so alone, try to recruit a close friend who has psychedelic experience to join you on your journey.

That said, tripping socially is more of an "outward" experience—which can be super fun and meaningful—but many experts would argue it's not exactly an inward-focused "healing" experience. However, for me, as someone with social anxiety, I find tripping in small groups to, in fact, be very healing because I can connect with people deeply without my usual reservation and anxiety. Plus, because of my increased sensitivity while under the influence of psychedelics, it can feel like I'm able to read my friends' minds and it helps me understand social situations more empathetically. However, on the other hand, tripping with others can get hectic, especially when the group is bigger than four or five people. What's more, should one person have a very challenging experience, it can affect the mood of the entire group negatively if it's not handled with care.

If your goal is to take mushrooms and "go inward" for personal growth or healing, then you might want to consider doing them on your own, preferably with a trip sitter. Tripping by yourself can be a profound learning experience, especially when you're able to close your eyes, listen to music, and let the journey take you where it feels you need to go. But this can also get very lonely, especially for those who struggle with feelings of isolation in everyday life. Some people swear by taking solo trips a couple of times a year to reconnect with themselves as a kind of emotional reset, but for the inexperienced user, this can be a bit challenging and possibly overwhelming or even frightening. So if you are considering this for your first psychedelic experience, definitely enlist a close friend or loved one to trip sit for you, and have them read Chapter 12 of this book to prepare!

HOW TO CREATE THE RIGHT SET

Preparing your mind-set is a little bit more difficult than your setting, but there are still some things to consider. First of all, it's normal to feel anticipation, excitement, or nervousness before your journey, but it's also crucial that you're relaxed. In fact, James Fadiman, author of *The Psychedelic Explorer's Guide* and prominent psychedelic researcher since the 1960s, recommends people take the entire day before a psychedelic experience to prepare and relax by spending time in nature, being reflective, and setting intentions for the upcoming psychedelic experience. If you can spare the time, this is a great way to prepare your set. If not, try to still spend a little time relaxing before ingesting your mushrooms by taking deep breaths, meditating, or doing some yoga. The point is to clear your mind and prepare it for its upcoming task: letting go to the psychedelic substance. So anything that you can do to center yourself before the journey will be helpful, as will approaching the experience with an accepting and open attitude rather than any sort of expectations. Basically, you have to be confident in yourself and your intentions and be open to any experiences that may arise—blissful or uncomfortable.

It's important to remember that set encompasses more than your feelings toward the experience and your mood the day of the trip, it also includes your underlying emotions, memories, beliefs, and your ability to release control. Remember that psychedelics can amplify your emotions, especially ones you've been trying to push down and not deal with. So if you've been depressed, anxious, suicidal, or struggling to grapple with some issue, there's a good chance psilocybin will bring you face-to-face with it. While these kinds of feelings aren't always known to us before going in, it's also important to closely evaluate how you're doing emotionally before taking a psychedelic, and figuring out if maybe it's the wrong time to trip.

But, when is a bad time to trip? I posed this question to my interviewees, and I got a bunch of interesting answers. For one, many people told me that if they were under a tremendous amount of stress, like in a lot of debt or had a lot of deadlines or responsibilities, it was a bad time to take a psychedelic. Others mentioned receiving deeply emotional news, such as a loved one having cancer, as being a bad time to trip. I would also say from experience that if you are feeling suicidal or struggling with a lot of self-hatred, it can be a difficult time to trip. Even though in clinical trials psilocybin is having a lot of preliminary success in treating depression, if you do mushrooms on your own in the midst of occasional suicidal ideation, tripping can amplify that feeling without any of the positive effects like catharsis or transcendence. It's not that you're too damaged to do mushrooms, but you should be in a more secure headspace because your thoughts can turn against you and become somewhat delusional or overbearing while tripping. If you're not sure how depressed or stable you are, it's a good reason to enlist a professional guide to give you the extra support you may need.

SETTING PREPARATION TIPS

The importance of choosing and planning for the right set and setting cannot be understated. More so than the dose or the type of drug itself, your set and setting will have the greatest influence over your trip. As I learned as a teenager, buying a bag of shrooms in a parking lot and shoving them down right away is not the way to have a safe and meaningful psychedelic experience. Planning and preparation are key, but everyone has their own preferences, routine, and ritual. Likely, your perfect set and setting will be a trial-and-error process, as you learn which things you like and don't while in that sensitive state of mind. Yet, there are some crucial things to consider, including any supplies and provisions you may need, so let's break them down.

LOCATION

We've already gone through the importance of a comfortable and supportive setting for your psychedelic experience, but let's talk about logistics. Where should you actually trip?

First of all, you need to decide if you want to have your journey indoors or outside. Inside is definitely the safest option with the least amount of potential interruptions—which is great for going inward—but having a psychedelic journey outdoors can be magical. In a safe, familiar, and secluded outdoor setting, psychedelics have been known to induce feelings of oneness or unity with nature, which can have profound, lasting effects on one's life and how you see and connect with the rest of the world. It's a common experience to realize we humans are not separate from nature but an integral part of it, and that has also prompted many to begin taking better care of the environment following their trip. However, you still need to prepare for all the unpredictable factors of an outdoor journey, like insects, animals, weather, and the possibility of seeing other people. Remember to bring and apply things like sunscreen and insect repellent before you start tripping and make a plan for other possible situations.

The best solution? If it's possible, plan a psychedelic experience in a place where you can go both indoors and out. Ideally, you want to trip in a house with a big backyard or garden so you have the comfort of being inside, but have the option of going outdoors somewhere safe and private. Back in the sixties, during the heyday of original psychedelic therapy, many therapists preferred to give patients the psychedelic substance in a comfortable indoor setting—typically a room in a university decorated to look like a living room. Then, after the peak of the experience, they would offer participants the chance to go outside on a nature walk with their facilitators.[78] This way, participants were indoors "going inward" during the most intense part of the journey, then, they could go outside and appreciate nature while they were still feeling the effects but were slowly coming down.

---

78   Richards, *Sacred Knowledge: Psychedelics and Religious Experiences.*

Many people choose to stay home for their trips, and that's perfectly okay too. Even if you live in a cramped apartment, home might be the place where you feel the safest, so that's your best bet, especially for your first trip. In fact, many of the mushroom users I interviewed told me they prefer to take mushrooms at home, but they each had their own conditions and routines. To prepare, the most common thing people told me they do is to clean their house. It sounds kind of weird, but there's something about tripping among mess and clutter that can turn people's experiences sour. So sweep the floor, wipe down the kitchen and bathroom, do whatever you need to make your house feel tidy, and it can make a big difference.

If you have roommates whom you won't be sharing the experience with, consider picking a day or night for your trip when they won't be home. If you're close and you don't feel judged by them, it might not matter. But as we discussed earlier, the presence of other people, especially those not "on the medicine," can greatly affect your experience. You want the environment to feel supportive, so if your roommates are your close friends who hold space for you all the time, then make sure you communicate what you'll be doing beforehand. But if you don't feel supported by your housemates or you're not very close, it may be in your best interest to find a six-to-eight-hour block of time when they're not home to take your mushroom journey.

What I would recommend against, especially if this is your first time trying mushrooms, is going to a public park or event where there will be lots of people. This can be stress inducing rather than relaxing. You might find yourself trying to hide the fact that you're "on drugs" or wondering if everyone can tell. Plus, talking to strangers while you're on a psychedelic can be a very disconcerting experience. I would also recommend against camping out in the middle of nowhere for your first trip because of its lack of creature comforts and just in case you need emergency assistance or support. Yet, for a more experienced user and at an appropriate dose (low to moderate), bringing some mushrooms along for a camping trip can be a magical experience.

The main takeaway? Give your location some consideration and do what feels right. Remember, being comfortable both physically and emotionally are the most important things when choosing the right place to trip on mushrooms.

MUSIC AND LIGHTING

The right music and lighting can make or break a psychedelic experience. They really establish the mood for your setting, and so they have a huge impact on your entire trip. But it can be hard to know what music and lighting you'll prefer before you start tripping, so let me offer a few suggestions.

For many, music is a crucial component of their mushroom journey. Yet choosing a song or album to put on while you're tripping can be really difficult, as I learned recently from experience. I was really overwhelmed by my iTunes collection and turned off by a lot of my options, and so I couldn't decide on what music to listen to. Your best bet is to prepare a playlist before you eat your mushrooms. You may even want to make a few different playlists to invoke different moods, like happy, introspective, calm, or trippy. That way, if you start to get sick of your music selection or feel it doesn't fit your mood, you can just select a new playlist rather than trying to find a new album, artist, or song. Also make your playlists long so you can just leave them on for hours and not worry too much about DJing. And be sure to download your playlists and make them available offline before you eat your mushrooms so you can leave your phone on airplane mode during your trip.

But what kind of music do you choose for a psychedelic experience? That's a great question, and there are a couple of things to consider. For one, many people find that they end up enjoying music they would never listen to regularly. Things like tribal drumming or classical symphonies can really work while you're tripping, even if you'd never listen to that kind of thing during your commute to work. Lots of people enjoy ambient, electronic music that can also include sounds from nature like birds chirping or water trickling.

Another thing to consider is that the music you listen to can affect your emotional state. For instance, if you listen to a really sad song, or one that reminds you of your ex or your mother, that can have a profound impact on your set. That's not to say you should only listen to "happy" music, but it may be a reason to avoid music with words or emotional significance. It's totally up to you, and some people seek out songs with emotional significance on purpose for that same reason. It'll depend on your intentions for the trip and the mood you want to set. If you're still stumped on what music to listen to, check out the "Listening" section at the end of this book!

Lighting also affects your experience, although to a less emotional degree. Because your eyes are more sensitive to brightness and your visual field will likely be distorted, you'll want dim yet warm and inviting lighting. For example, I recently moved into a new house, and the first time I took mushrooms here, I didn't want to spend a lot of time in my bedroom because it was too dark and uninviting. To be fair, my bedroom is a dark blue color, but I didn't realize it would be an issue before I started my trip. For my next journey, I put white Christmas lights above the bed and set up the TV with a trippy Spotify playlist before eating my mushrooms. The lights and music made a huge difference; I spent most of my trip in that space enjoying the ambience, watching geometrical shapes dance around the shadows and textures of my ceiling, and having deep insights about myself and my work. So always set up mood lighting and music beforehand and continue to look for ways you can improve your setup for the next trip.

TIMING

Because a mushroom trip lasts around six hours, you want to plan the timing of your experience. For instance, you'll have to decide if you'd prefer to trip during the day or night, or perhaps a little bit of both. It's really a personal preference, and it will probably also depend on whether you're tripping indoors or out. For an outdoor trip on a low to moderate dose, I personally like to take them before midday so I can spend my whole trip outside, watching the sunlight reflect off the leaves and just enjoying all of my senses. But for an inward-focused, higher-dose journey, I prefer to take them at home in the late afternoon, around 4:00 or 5:00 p.m. That way I peak around sunset, and finish tripping around 10:00 p.m., so I can still get a full night's sleep.

Yet, many people like to take their mushrooms at night, like one of my interviewees, cannabis writer William Sumner. He told me he likes to eat his mushrooms around 10:00 p.m. and trip through the night, watching the sunrise to come down and end his experience. His reasoning was pretty straightforward: No one's trying to get in touch with him at that time, and so he feels the most comfortable relinquishing his control to the magic fungi. In the past, a call from his parents during a daytime trip set him off into a paranoid, negative thought loop he'd prefer not to repeat.

Taking mushrooms around midnight and tripping throughout the night is also how they are taken ceremoniously in traditional indigenous cultures in Mexico.[79] The late Terence McKenna, author, speaker, and famous psychonaut, recommended people take a heroic dose (5 grams) in a dark, quiet room, without other stimulations or distractions. He felt that's how mushrooms taught people the most about themselves and the universe, and his famous saying "Sit down, shut up, and pay attention" reflects this advice. But taking a moderate dose of around 2 to 3 grams and wearing an eye mask at any hour could still produce similar results at a more manageable intensity.

Another important thing to mention is that mushrooms can make people tired the next day, especially if they kept you up late or you fasted before eating them. So take it into consideration before heading straight to work the following morning. If you work a regular nine-to-five job, I would suggest taking the mushrooms on Saturday and relaxing on Sunday, or even planning to trip during a three-day weekend. In fact, many of the users I spoke to also told me they try to set aside two to three days for a mushroom trip. It's not so much that mushrooms give you some kind of hangover, but the experiences they elicit can be powerful, and it can be difficult to go back to the real world,

79 Schultes, et al., *Plants of the Gods.*

especially work, the following day. To get the most benefit out of your trip, it's best to relax the next day and reflect on your experience. While integration takes place over the course of the following weeks, months, and even years, the day after a trip is a crucial time to reflect and journal while the experience is still fresh.

ACTIVITIES AND SUPPLIES

If you think that the mushrooms are your activity and supplies, you're not totally wrong, but because psilocybin is so stimulating, it can be fun to have things around that engage your different senses. For example, Ashley Manta told me she likes to have various textured fabrics and blankets around, especially really soft and cozy things, to touch and to engage her partner with. Manta also told me she likes to have different lights and pretty things for her and her friends to look at. She even bought a special trippy lamp on Amazon for about 15 dollars specifically to enhance her mushroom journeys.

Many people report having art supplies and paper around for their trips, even if they don't consider themselves artists in the "default world." Making art can be a fun, tactile experience, sometimes full of significance even if your masterpiece doesn't look like much the next day. Plus, because mushrooms make many people feel like a kid again they can also lower inhibitions or self-judgment in regard to making art, and you can just see where the paint or crayon takes you. Speaking of crayons, Rachelle Gordon, writer and director of strategic partnerships, told me she enjoys using adult coloring books while she's tripping. She even has a specific coloring book that she adds to while she's on mushrooms that's become its own trip journal of sorts. But you can get creative and plan what feels right. Maybe you want to make or buy some play dough beforehand or have some Legos to build with. The key is setting everything up before you start the experience because it can seem a bit overwhelming to dig out the toys or art supplies while you're feeling the mushrooms. Set up an area of your house for art or play, like the kitchen table or living room, and venture over when you're in the mood for an activity.

Keeping a journal around is also a super common supply for a psychedelic experience. Drawing and recording insights can be an important part of a mushroom trip and really interesting to look over afterward. Just be sure not to hold yourself back too much by recording every single sensation you have or you might be missing some of the experience.

For musicians and the non-musically inclined alike, playing with instruments and other ways to make sound can be really fun on mushrooms too. Guitars and drums are popular options, as are more simple instruments like shakers, bongos, or tambourines. These kinds of percussive instruments can also be good for releasing energy and working through some difficult emotions or memories that may arise. Just be careful not to wake up your whole neighborhood if you decide to trip during the middle of the night!

When you're starting to come down, you may crave doing something normal to ground yourself and relax, like watching your favorite series. But regular TV and movies can seem kind of weird while the mushrooms are still in your system. So, another tip is to download some nature documentaries before you start tripping, like *Planet Earth* or anything else narrated by David

Attenborough. Nature docs can be tantalizing and a great way to transition back to reality and enjoy the beauty and awesomeness of Mother Nature. They can also be an engaging way to distract yourself from overly negative thoughts if you get stuck in a challenging place and can't work through it.

In clinical trials with psilocybin, participants are usually given an eye mask, headphones with music, and a blanket for their trip. Although using mushrooms on your own is different than in a research setting, an eye mask and headphones can really help you eliminate distractions and focus on going inward. If you're curious to try, simply close your eyes with or without listening to music, and relax, taking deep breaths. For many, their visuals and insights are the most intense with eyes closed, so it's definitely worth giving it a try if you're curious.

If you do plan on going inward—or even if you're not—I would recommend having some tissues or soft toilet paper around. For many, myself most definitely included, crying can be a big part of the psilocybin experience. It's not necessarily always sad tears, although often sad things will bubble up that I haven't been dealing with. Sometimes I'll cry for the sheer beauty of things or for the deep connection or appreciation I feel for the person I'm tripping with or thinking about. But if they are sad tears, they're not necessarily bad. In fact, crying on mushrooms can be one of the most cathartic experiences of your life, so if you feel the tears coming on, don't fight them, just reach for the tissues.

Another thing researchers since the 1960s have been bringing to psychedelic sessions are freshly cut flowers, especially roses. Staring at a rosebud has helped many people on psychedelics come to profound realizations as well as promoted incredible visuals like that of the flower blooming or dying, depending on your thought process. Flowers can be especially lovely to have around if you're planning on spending your entire psychedelic experience indoors, because they invoke some of that connectedness to nature many people cherish while on mushrooms. They can also be useful if you're having a challenging experience or get stuck in a negative thought loop. Like the other activities and supplies we mentioned, staring at a flower can also help get you out of a challenging place or distract you from paranoid or overly negative thoughts. Other decorative things can work the same way, like crystals, art or nature books, textiles, and mandalas. So even if they're not a regular decoration in your space, hang some up or put some out beforehand and go seek them out when you're feeling anxious, sad, or bored.

FOOD

In terms of food, you've probably heard that you won't be very hungry during your mushroom trip, but there's actually a bit you can do to prepare to make your journey as successful as possible. First of all, during the week leading up to your trip, try to eat and sleep as well as you can. It can also be beneficial to avoid a lot of processed food during that time, but that's not completely necessary.

For the day of your trip, it's best not to eat too much at all before ingesting the mushrooms. While some recommend fasting completely, I would be wary of this technique if it's your first trip because it can make the mushrooms kick in faster and stronger. If you're planning on tripping during the day, I would recommend eating a light, healthy breakfast first. Eggs, toast, and fruit would be perfect or a veggie omelet and a side of fruit, basically something wholesome and nutritious. You also may want to just opt for some fruit if you plan on eating the mushrooms early in the day.

The reason you don't want to stuff yourself with a huge meal or two first is because that can increase your chance of nausea during your trip. If you plan on taking psilocybin in the evening, have a regular healthy breakfast and then a light lunch or consider only having fruit and bread for lunch. It'll depend on what time you're taking the mushrooms, but the important thing is to avoid taking them on a completely full or totally empty stomach. I personally like to eat a light meal and then fast for three or four hours before I drink my mushrooms in a tea (see page 76). It's also important to mention that you might want to avoid super spicy or acidic foods the day of your trip because it could contribute to some indigestion.

While you likely won't be hungry during your trip, it can be nice to have some snacks in the house, like fresh fruit, to eat while you're tripping. Because all of your senses can feel so enhanced and different, it can be a real treat to bite into a juicy mango, strawberry, watermelon—or whatever your favorite fruits are. Experiencing different textures while you're tripping can also be fun, so consider buying a variety of snacks the day before. Just remember to cut up fruits like pineapple or mango before you begin your journey and save them in a container in the fridge. I also honestly like to buy some junk food, like potato chips or pretzels and chocolates. You probably won't be super drawn to consuming too much, but having some different things around to experiment with can be a real treat.

It's also important to have lots of purified water around, and it can be super refreshing to have a nice cold glass of ice water while you're tripping. Because of the enhanced sensations, it can be fun to have different drinks around to experiment with. Drinking bubbly soda can be a whole adventure on its own as it tickles the nose, as can some refreshing fruit juice or coconut water. Many people also like to have a cup of herbal tea during the experience—just don't forget you have the kettle on! I like to have some nice beer in the house for afterward, but that's also just a personal preference.

If you're concerned you may feel nauseous during your trip, many find it helpful to have different ginger products along for the ride. It can be ginger ale, tea, or candies—whatever you prefer. Ginger can help settle the stomach and also give you peace of mind if you're worried nausea will be your dominating sensation. If you've tried mushrooms before and you struggled to keep them down, you may want to consider making them into a tea (see sidebar).

In preparation, experienced mushroom users also like to have everything at home for a nice meal or snack after the mushrooms have worn off. People can be really particular regarding what they like to eat after psilocybin, but your body might crave something sort of wholesome. For some, that means buying a fancy frozen pizza, but for others, it might mean a nice vegetarian soup. It's likely you'll be too pooped to cook, but it also might be too soon to go out in public to grab something. So having something pre-made or frozen that you can heat up is helpful. Many people's stomachs still feel a bit too off to eat much of anything, but it's better to have some food around rather than forcing yourself to go out after a potentially heavy experience. Of course, ordering delivery is also an option if the trip ends at a reasonable hour and a member of your party doesn't mind opening the door!

How to Make Magic Mushroom Tea

1. Weigh out your dose of dried mushrooms.

2. Blitz the mushrooms up into a powder in a blender, food processor, or coffee grinder.

3. Peel and cut up some pieces of raw ginger.

4. Pour hot water over powdered mushrooms and ginger.

5. Wait 10 to 15 minutes.

6. Add honey to taste.

7. Drink the tea and then eat all the remaining mushroom bits! It can help to pour some cold water in your cup to finish it all off.

OTHER SETTING CONSIDERATIONS

Just a few last considerations before we move on to set. First of all, the right setting is more than the right place with the right people, it's the right place set up well. So that means cleaning as well as making it look welcoming and trip-friendly, whether that's putting fresh flowers in each room, setting up your kitchen with activities or art supplies, hanging trippy lights in the bedroom, or all of the above. Pretend the mushrooms are your honored guests and you have to prepare the house for their presence. For me, preparing also includes setting up music in each room of my house so I don't have to deal with any technical electronic stuff when I'm actually tripping.

For a friend of mine from college, it also means setting up "nesting spots" around the house. Basically, she makes sure each room is stocked with plenty of blankets and pillows before each trip so she and her partner have places to cuddle and talk, as well as to build forts. She told me that because she feels so much like a kid again on mushrooms, building forts and then relaxing in them is a highlight of her at-home psychedelic experiences. I also do something similar, where I just make sure each room of my house has cozy places to sit and lounge. For me, that also means making sure there's dry furniture in my outdoor spaces; I'll also hang up a hammock in my patio and leave some yoga mats outside to lie on and look at the stars after the sun goes down.

Another key consideration is turning off your phone or putting it on airplane mode. It's not that you'll crave going on Instagram while tripping; in fact, social media can seem kind of weird. But you don't want an unexpected phone call or text message stressing you out. If you have certain people you're in regular contact with, tell them the day before your trip that you'll be offline for about eight hours and you'll get in touch when you have service again. You don't have to tell them exactly what you're doing, but you can if they're open to psychedelics; totally up to you and whatever makes you feel the most comfortable.

Lastly, for my readers who enjoy joints or hand-rolled cigarettes while they're tripping (no judgment), I would recommend you roll up before the experience begins. Cannabis can be a very interesting yet intense addition to a mushroom trip. More on this combination in Chapter 14, but if you do plan on mixing the two, get it all prepared first. Grinding up weed and rolling a joint (or tobacco cigarette) can be difficult and take ages while you're tripping. Plus, your fingers can jam up and the whole process can seem overwhelming, so roll a few up beforehand and you'll be all set.

MINDSET PREPARATION SUGGESTIONS

Preparing your mind-set for a psychedelic experience can be a little more difficult than the setting, but there are some ways to center yourself and create an open and relaxed attitude before you dive in.

INTENTIONS

Setting intentions for your psilocybin trip can be extremely easy or very difficult. Intentions are what you hope to get from the trip, what you hope to learn, or why you're taking mushrooms. They can be simple like, "I'm curious to see what the mushrooms will show me" or more personal like "I'd like to learn how to forgive my father." If you're taking mushrooms with close friends, family members, or loved ones, your intentions could be to connect with those people on a deeper level. Everyone has their own intentions when taking psilocybin, and very often, the mushrooms will provide you with an experience that is completely different—causing many dedicated psilonauts to declare: "the mushrooms had intentions of their own."

Setting intentions can be beneficial, especially if you want to use mushrooms for healing. However, intentions can also be unhelpful if you're too focused on them or if you set too many. When I interviewed experienced mushroom users for this book, only about half told me they set intentions at all. But most of them had the same reason for not setting any: They've learned to just accept the experience the mushrooms give them and they've stopped trying to direct it to their own prerogatives. It's great advice because it's when you try to rein in mushrooms too tightly that you're more likely to get anxiety or succumb to a challenging trip.

Yet, intention setting can also be a good way to center yourself and relax before a journey. Think about your intentions and explore them by journaling. Then, choose a simple and honest phrase and write it down on a small piece of paper and place it on your altar, if you've made one. I've found this practice to be more helpful than going into a psychedelic experience with a laundry list of complicated goals, then my trips tend to be more challenging and complicated as well. But when I set a simple, direct intention, like "I want to love myself" or "Teach me. I'm listening," then I've had more meaningful and less overwhelming experiences. While my setting and preparation are also huge factors, I believe my intentions have had a major influence on the direction of my trips. The key is centering yourself on a fairly basic idea and being able to come back to it for support. So try to set a simple and honest intention by writing it down beforehand and see what happens.

CREATING YOUR OWN RITUAL OR CEREMONY

In the psychedelic community, ceremonies are often spoken of as a creating a "container" for a psychedelic journey because without ritual, it can be difficult to process such a powerful life event. Therefore, you can prepare your mind-set by crafting your own ceremony for your mushroom trip. Your ritual could be anything; it could be simply mindfully drinking a tea that contains mushrooms and ginger or more advanced like making an altar, saying a prayer, and burning sage. The important thing is, you're signaling to yourself that you are doing something with intent, says Amanda Schendel, founder of the psilocybin retreat The Buena Vida, which practices shamanic ceremony. If that speaks to you, come up with your own ceremony or ritual to honor and signify the experience.

If you're interested in making an altar as part of your own personal ceremony, there's no wrong way to do it. Many people set aside a space in their homes and decorate it with items of significance, like photos of loved ones or rocks from places they've been, as well as offerings to the earth and plant spirits, and religious or spiritual symbols. You can also include your written intentions, flowers, crystals, incense, even significant foods if you want to. Some people like to leave the mushrooms they're about to eat on their altar the day before their trip to honor their power. Others choose their favorite lipstick, book, or a lucky pair of underwear—there's no right or wrong way to make an altar so don't be intimidated if you've never made one before.

JOURNAL

Journaling before, after, and even during your experience can be a great way to get the most out of your trip. It can be very helpful in preparing the right set and exploring your feelings preceding a psychedelic experience. Try journaling not only right before the trip, but a whole week before or more if you can. Explore your fears and anxieties about the upcoming journey: What do you hope to learn or see? Do you want to learn more about yourself, connect with nature, or your spouse? Or maybe you have no idea what your intentions are other than curiosity about mushrooms. That's okay too. Journal about it anyway and you might find that there's more there than you originally anticipated.

DO YOUR HOMEWORK

An easy way to prepare your mind-set is by doing your homework. Reading this book is an excellent start, but consider checking out other books on psychedelics, both their therapeutic potential and other users' first-person accounts. There's a ton of information online, like forums on Reddit, Erowid, and similar sites, as well as articles and publications on psychedelics. There are also documentary films and podcasts about psychedelics, as well as other related topics like altered states of consciousness, mystical experiences, and transpersonal psychology. Devouring psychedelic media can help you prepare for a wide range of possible experiences and outcomes, and it can also help you make sense of your trip after the fact. Be sure to check out the "Further Reading, Viewing, and Listening" section at the end of this book for more resources!

HYGIENE AND CLOTHES

This one may seem obvious—of course you'll have a shower and get dressed before tripping—but throughout my interviews with mushrooms users, I learned many people have whole personal-care routines they like to go through before embarking on a mushroom journey. For example, Sarah ElSayed, cannabis publicist, brand strategist, and founder of Grass is Greener PR, told me she likes to get ready as if she's going out, by doing her full makeup and hair, even though she typically stays in her apartment to trip. Her reasoning was simple—if she looks in the mirror during the journey, she wants to like what she sees. She explained she started this ritual after tripping once without doing so, and when she got a glimpse of herself in the mirror, it was a negative experience. So if you're the kind of person who enjoys getting done up and prefers the way you look with makeup, don't skip that step on trip day.

For me, someone who doesn't wear a lot of makeup, I just like to make sure I'm clean and comfortable. So I'll take a nice hot shower beforehand, brush my teeth thoroughly, do the rest of my personal care routine, and I'm good to go. If I had a bathtub at my house and was doing an evening trip, I might take a nice hot bath beforehand, giving myself time to relax and get in the right headspace first.

One thing I definitely recommend is wearing loose, comfortable clothes. Mushrooms can change your sense of body temperature, so having different layers and therefore options for hot or cold, no matter the season, is a must. I'd also recommend having a warm blanket you can snuggle under, even if it's the middle of the summer. I recently tripped on mushrooms in the jungle, and although it was over 80 degrees Fahrenheit and humid, I still felt myself getting chilly and wanting to put on my hoodie and cuddle under a blanket. At the same time, others with me felt very hot and sweaty, so having options around is helpful to make sure you're always physically comfortable.

BABYSITTER

Different from getting a "trip sitter," this time I mean an actual babysitter for children if you're a parent. I've had a couple of different parents recently tell me they don't like tripping. When I asked them why, they both told me stories of bad trips, where they felt really terrible about themselves and their parenting skills. But in both cases, it was because they were tripping around their children. Before you get up in arms, in both of these cases one of the parents was on psychedelics while their spouse stayed sober to care for the kids, but it still turned out negatively for the tripping partner. Both people who told me about this experience reported feeling incredibly irresponsible for using such a powerful substance around their kids, feeling completely incapable of parenting under the influence, and this resulted in an anxious and challenging experience.

If you're a parent, this doesn't mean you can't use mushrooms occasionally, but I would highly suggest getting a babysitter for the duration of your experience. And if your kids can stay the night at a friend's or family member's house, that would be ideal. When you're under the influence of psychedelics, your kids might sense you're acting different, and you won't be able to care for them at the same level, especially if an emergency arises. But I also highly recommend getting a babysitter so you can have the best and most beneficial experience. With your children around, even if there's a sober adult watching them for you, you won't be able to let go completely and embrace the psychedelic experience. Instead you'll likely be fighting it and trying to act normal, which is not fun and a recipe for a bad or anxious trip. So save yourself the grief and plan ahead by booking a babysitter or asking a family member to watch the kids for at least the six to eight hours that the mushrooms are actively in your system.

INTEGRATION PREP

While journaling is great integration prep, there are a couple of other things you can do before your trip to help you prepare to integrate. For one, talking about your experience is going to help, so think about the people in your life who will be open to hearing about your insights under the influence of a stigmatized and likely illegal substance. Friends and family with prior psychedelic experience will be helpful because they'll have more of a framework to understand where you're coming from.

Another great option is to look up psychedelic support groups in your area. These are typically free meetups of 15 to 30 people who have recently had psychedelic journeys they want to talk about. They're a great place to openly share your experience without feeling judged or stigmatized, especially if you've had a challenging trip or are having difficulty adjusting back to your everyday life. If you'd like professional support through this process, an option you might want to consider is finding a therapist who specializes in psychedelic integration. These are not underground therapists who provide guided trips, but instead, aboveground social workers and psychologists who help people prepare for and unpack psychedelic experiences. They won't judge you for using substances, but they also won't help you find any either. However, if you plan to do some serious healing with psilocybin or had a really troubling experience that's hard to make sense of, they can be a great source of support. More on integration and these professionals in Chapter 11.

The last way to prepare your set is to realize you might feel a bit stirred up after your trip. "People may be experiencing things that they were shut down to. They may have had really profound insights that are going to generate a lot of positive change. But there's a period of adjusting to knowing this new material. And that can be quite unsettling in an overall good way," explains psychedelic integration specialist Elizabeth Nielson. Basically, don't be surprised if you feel a wide range of emotions, both positive and negative, in the days and weeks following your psychedelic experience. "It's par for the course and it's okay," says Nielson. "As long as there's care around it and compassion toward it and acceptance of it. And the curiosity about it that leads to it being integrated in a productive way."

This all may seem like a lot to do for a six-hour drug experience, but trust me and all the seasoned users I talked to when I tell you it's worth it. When you've fully prepared your set and setting, you'll be more likely to let go to the substance and have a meaningful trip. And remember, all these ideas are just suggestions—do what feels right to you and tweak as you become more experienced.

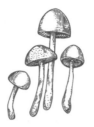

Chapter 6

GUIDED TRIPS

If your interest in mushrooms lies in the desire to heal, doing them alone at home is more difficult and often less effective than with a guide, sitter, shaman, at a retreat, or as a participant in a clinical trial. Let's go through all of your options to break down the pros and cons so you can choose the best level of support for you and your goals.

RETREATS

There are retreats for everything nowadays, from yoga and meditation to darkness and even silence retreats, that offer people the chance to take a week or so from their busy lives and focus solely on themselves. Psilocybin mushroom retreats also offer people that chance, and they can combine many of the other life skills, like yoga and meditation, if you want. At the time of writing this book, mushroom retreats are still very new and available only in a handful of countries with lax mushroom laws, like Jamaica, the Netherlands, and Mexico. Therefore, these retreats operate mostly legally and can be the easiest way to do mushrooms in a safe, supportive environment. That being said, psychedelic retreats can be expensive and so aren't financially feasible for everyone. Hopefully, as psychedelic awareness spreads and grows, costs will eventually change.

Compared to doing mushrooms at home, especially for your first time, retreats offer the safety of trained and experienced facilitators to be there if things get rough or scary. That alone can provide people the peace of mind to let go more easily and embrace the experience. They also offer the security of a measured dose and trusted source of mushrooms, which obviously has its perks. But retreat experiences can vary greatly, so how do you choose the one that's right for you?

Group retreats are a popular choice in the ayahuasca community, and that trend is now extending to mushrooms. I recently attended a weeklong group ceremonial mushroom retreat that was exactly the experience I needed, even though I was terrified in the weeks leading up to it. I consider myself seriously introverted and struggle to put myself out there and form connections with new people. So while the thought of the group experience made me sweat, I also hoped it could help me loosen up and learn how to connect with people again. Amanda Schendel told me over the phone that nearly everyone who comes to The Buena Vida retreats considers themself an introvert with social anxiety. I laughed out loud, "That's me!" The group experience definitely opened my eyes to a lot of things about myself that helped me start to heal my social anxiety. For instance, the damage in constantly comparing myself to other people became very clear, and the reality that we're all dealing with tough issues—I'm not the most damaged person in the world—was an eye-opener. It helped me realize the importance of community and how I can isolate myself unnecessarily. A group retreat was also beneficial for my integration. Being able to discuss my trips with the whole group the mornings after, and reaching out to those people in the form of a massive group text if things get tough, or if I'm particularly proud of something, continues to be valuable.

While many psychedelic retreats are groups, one of the ways The Buena Vida stands out is that it offers psilocybin sessions in the form of three shamanic ceremonies of incremental doses. The ceremony was based on indigenous tradition, with a shaman leading the group's experience. For most of the six hours, she sang both traditional healing songs from a variety of native cultures as well as more modern tunes, like "Somewhere Over the Rainbow." She had an incredible voice and was a trained jazz singer, but she also utilized sound healing instruments to really elevate the whole experience to an unearthly level. Not all retreats take ritual as seriously, and from what I've heard, others instead give everyone psilocybin capsules together and have facilitators watch over them for safety and support, without a shaman present. This may be fine for some people, but for me, the ceremony helped me to honor the mushrooms' power and to learn my own.

For me, the ceremony and group integration meetings coupled with the yoga and meditation classes, sound therapy, acupuncture, and healthy vegetarian food helped to not only make sense of my experience but to allow me to experiment with ways to integrate those lessons once I got back home. It was the full self-care package, with psilocybin mushrooms as the psychedelic cherry on top.

The retreat I attended was co-ed, but there are also women's-only and men's-only retreats popping up, and I believe other variations will emerge as well. The most important thing when picking a retreat is making sure it's safe and you'll be comfortable there. For me, knowing The Buena Vida was founded and run by women made me feel safe, and after talking to Schendel on the phone for almost an hour before signing up, I felt confident that tripping with them would make me feel secure and supported. Plus, I read through their past guest reviews thoroughly, which I also suggest you do on sites like Retreat Guru.[80] So, when choosing a retreat, don't sign up for the first one you see, but do your homework and pick the experience and group of people that make you feel the safest. For a more detailed safety checklist of ways to research a psychedelic retreat, check out "20 Safety Tips for Those Participating in Ceremonies That Use Psychoactive Substances" on the Women's Visionary Congress website.[81]

GUIDE, SHAMAN, OR TRIP SITTER?

Guides, shamans, trip sitters—their jobs aren't much different, except each may provide more or less support in the days before and after your trip. Yet, they can have so many different titles and work almost exclusively underground and thus can be tricky

---

80   Retreat Guru. https://retreat.guru

81   Women's Visionary Congress. https://www.visionarycongress.org/safety-tips-for-participating-in-psychedelic-ceremonies

to locate and research. How do you know which type to choose and trust?

A psychedelic guide can have a variety of credentials. Some are actual therapists (think psychologists or clinical social workers) that work privately with plant medicine and may have even trained with Stanislav Grof or his predecessors.[82] But that's not always the case. Many psychedelic guides don't have advanced degrees in psychology but have done extensive research and plant medicine work on their own, and they feel compelled to share that knowledge with others. There are also people who call themselves shamans, many of whom have trained with indigenous groups in places like South America, and they may provide more ceremony or spirituality to the experience, but of course, that is not guaranteed. However, it can be hard to vet people like this or even locate them at all, and, unfortunately, there are accounts of people being abused by underground psychedelic guides and shamans in their own cities and abroad at retreats.[83, 84] So be careful and thorough when investigating guides in your area: meet them in person first, talk to some of their previous clients if possible, and make sure you feel totally comfortable with the person before entering a psychedelic experience with them.

Then, of course, there are trip sitters, which may be the easiest and least expensive version for people. Trip sitters can be anyone, especially someone you trust unconditionally, like a close friend, partner, or family member, if they're open to the

---

82   According to Michael Pollan's book, *How to Change Your Mind* (2018), beginning in 1973, Grof trained hundreds of psychotherapists "who wanted to incorporate psychedelics in their practices. Many if not most of the therapists and guides now doing this work underground learned their craft at the feet of Stan Grof in the Big House at Esalen" (pg. 45).

83   MacLean, "Psychedelic Ethics: The Good, the Bad, and the Ugly."

84   Monroe, Rachel. "Sexual Assault in the Amazon."

idea. It's good to ask a friend with some psychedelic experience, but not totally necessary. They essentially just need to have the time (at least six hours) to come and be a calm supportive presence that keeps you safe while you enter an altered state of consciousness. As far as the difference between guides and sitters, trip sitters are typically a little less involved than guides, especially in the days before and after your experience. I would say another distinction is that guides are more likely to have training of some kind, but nowadays, that might not be the case. For instance, the Zendo Project, a nonprofit organization that provides psychedelic peer support at music festivals and hosts trip-sitting training weekends, and other organizations are hosting trip-sitting classes around the US as well, so sitters are not necessarily untrained. On the other hand, not all guides are trained; especially because most of this work has been illegal for so long, there's no certificate or regulations at the moment, so it can be a fuzzy area to navigate. However, if you have a friend willing to trip sit but they have no experience, training isn't really necessary, just patience; a kind, open heart; and reading Chapter 12 of this book! Not everyone is going to require the high level of support that guides can offer, and for many, a trip sitter will be more than enough to help them have a safe and meaningful journey. The bottom line: do your homework and see what feels right.

There is one other guided trip option, which is more legal and easier to find information about. Some guides have begun hosting one-on-one psilocybin sessions in countries where mushrooms are more legal, like Jamaica and Mexico. It's the same idea as a retreat, where you fly to another country to take mushrooms, but many are just one-day private sessions rather than weeklong group vacations. Joe Moore and Kyle Buller, cofounders of *Psychedelics Today*, are beginning to offer these legal psilocybin sessions abroad catering to those who want to do mushrooms for healing legally in a one-on-one environment. Based on the "Johns Hopkins model" (basically the psychedelic therapy model we discuss in Chapter 3), participants will only stay one night to do one guided session. By wearing an eye mask and headphones, trippers will be encouraged to go inward and let the mushrooms bring up what they will in a "non-directive" approach, emphasizing the individual's own "inner-healing intelligence," Moore tells me over the phone. Sessions are preceded by a three-hour video-chat preparatory session and followed by another few video calls, access to Psychedelics Today's online courses, community message boards, and integration workbook and journal. Their goal is to provide a high level of support, which could be necessary for those who want to work on more difficult or trauma-based issues, or who may be overwhelmed or distracted by a group experience.

In general, having a guide or trip sitter can really help to keep you safe, physically and psychically. If you're considering doing mushrooms without any kind of support, just know that having a guide or sitter can not only help you feel more secure and comfortable "letting go" and "going deep," but tripping alone can also be a really lonely experience—having someone there, especially if you get hit with some really dark or powerful emotions, can be helpful. Plus, having the presence of a sober, supportive person to help with little things like music and people ringing the doorbell, to larger issues like any kind of emergency situation, can make all the difference. Especially for your first psychedelic experience or a high-dose trip, it's best not to go into it completely alone.

CLINICAL TRIALS

Of course, another option is applying to participate in a clinical trial using psilocybin. This is arguably the safest environment because it's the most well regulated and run by professionals with the most training and experience. At the moment, it also seems like participating in a clinical trial offers you the highest chance of a successful outcome. However, it's important to note that some trials use the double-blind method, meaning there's only a 50 percent chance that you'll receive psilocybin versus a placebo.[85] While not all trials are like this, you still need to qualify, which can be tricky in itself.

But the standard procedure for trials—psychedelic therapy—is a reason to pursue participating in one. I described it in depth in Chapter 3, but essentially you'll likely receive the highest level of interpersonal support in these trials, before, during, and after your psilocybin session(s). If and when psilocybin-assisted therapy becomes legal in the US, it will very likely follow this same protocol, and so it could eventually be available for people outside of the clinical trial context. Although there are some fears that this therapy will be very expensive and thus only

---

85   A large-scale, upcoming trial of psilocybin for treatment-resistant depression funded by the Usona Institute uses the double-blind method and so only 50 percent of participants receive psilocybin. This is a Phase II clinical trial to assess the safety and usefulness of psilocybin for major depressive disorder (MDD). Read more on their site: https://www.usonainstitute.org

accessible to a select number of wealthier individuals,[86] that still remains to be seen.

All in all, if you've decided you want a guide or sitter for your experience, the next step is to do your homework. See what's available in your area or in your budget. Once you've spoken with some guides, retreat leaders, or friends willing to trip sit, then listen to your intuition. What feels right? Who do you feel the safest with? Remember, feeling secure and comfortable with your guide is the most important factor when deciding between different options. If you're still not sure if you need a guide at all, really explore your reasons for taking mushrooms. For those looking to do some challenging inner work, having that extra support can really make a big difference in how your trip and integration play out.

---

86 Goldhill, "A Millionaire Couple Is Threatening."

Chapter 7

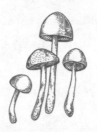

FINDING THE CORRECT DOSE

You've secured some mushrooms, but your source told you the whole bag will "get you there," so you should eat the entire thing, right? Wrong. Not when you're doing mushrooms mindfully like an adult! The correct dose is one of the most important aspects of having a safe trip, and figuring out the right dose for you can be tricky.

For one, when we talk about dose, we're typically referring to grams of dried psilocybin mushrooms (for fresh mushrooms, see Fresh Mushroom Dose Equivalent on page 96). However, even though we're going to use this measurement system in this chapter, it's important to discuss why it's flawed. Different types of mushrooms have different levels of psilocybin and psilocin, the psychoactive compounds that cause you to trip. Remember how there are over 180 different species of psilocybin-containing mushrooms? Similar to how different strains of cannabis vary in their strength and the experiences they produce, different types of mushrooms also have various intensities. While *Psilocybe cubensis* are the most common magic mushroom grown and sold, even different strains of this one species can vary in strength, like Golden Teachers, B+, and Penis Envy. Plus, how they were grown, dried, and stored also affects potency.

Fresh Mushroom Dose Equivalent

If you're planning on eating fresh mushrooms, finding an equivalent low, medium, and high dose will be a little different but still easy. Because fresh mushrooms are about 90 percent water, you need to multiply your desired dose by 10. So, if you'd like to try a moderate dose of 1.5 grams, you would need to eat 15 grams of fresh mushrooms.

Equation: (dried gram dose) x 10 = (wet gram dose)

Another reason why finding an ideal dose can be hard is that everyone reacts to mushrooms differently. This again rings true in regard to cannabis. If you pass a joint of the same weed around to five people, they could have five very different experiences. Well, the same is often true of mushrooms; even if you and five people take the same dose of the same batch of mushrooms, chances are you'll all have different experiences of varying intensities. Another thing to note is a person's weight or gender has very little to do with how mushrooms will affect them, so it's not really relevant to give heavier people more and lighter people less, for example.

What's more important with dosing is your prior experience with mushrooms and your set and setting, as described in Chapter 5. Previous experience with mushrooms or other classic psychedelics like LSD is important because in order to navigate high-dose trips safely and successfully, you need to get familiar with the psychedelic space and learn some tripping skills first. If you don't have any psychedelic experience, that's totally fine too. That's why I recommend starting at a fairly low dose and working your way up to a stronger one over the course of several trips.

Another thing to mention before we get into numbers is that different intentions and settings for your trip will also have different ideal doses. For example, if you're doing mushrooms with friends or your partner, and your intentions are to enhance your connection or to just have fun, you'll probably want to take a low to moderate dose. Whereas, if your intentions are healing, to lose your ego, feel a oneness with the universe, or elicit a spiritual experience, you'll want to take a higher dose once you've familiarized yourself with the psychedelic experience and developed some tripping skills. We'll get into this more as we describe recommended doses, but it's something to keep in mind as you read to consider the best dose for your desired experience.

FIRST TIME OR LOW DOSE

For your first time on a psychedelic or your first time in many years, I would highly recommend taking a low to moderate dose of between 0.5 and 2 grams of dried mushrooms. Like I mentioned above, tripping on higher doses requires some experience and navigation skills, which you can learn on a lower dose. At 0.5 to 2 grams, you will still be tripping, and could still have visuals and a ton of insight. In fact, depending on the strength of the mushrooms, 1.5 to 2 grams could still produce some of the higher-dose effects like ego loss or "oneness," especially if you're psychedelic-naïve, so it's important to get as much information about the fungi's strength you're about to ingest before doing so.

At the psilocybin retreat I attended recently, the facilitators and shaman gave participants a choice of consuming the same amount of mushrooms for our first ceremony: between 0.5 and 2 grams. I chose to take 1.5 grams because I had a bunch of psychedelic experience but hadn't taken mushrooms in a few years. At 1.5 grams I still had a very strong experience; it was incredibly emotional and physical. Even though it got dark and I had some suicidal thoughts, I was still very much aware of who and where I was (even if I hated both of them).

There's a big misconception that you should use a full eighth, 3.5 grams, for your first mushroom trip, but I and many of my interviewees, would advise against it. In fact, when I asked Mary Shock, tarot reader, collage artist, and healing work professional, what piece of advice she would give to a first-time tripper, she emphasized starting small and working your way to a higher dose over the course of years, if you need to. Her reasoning? She learned from experience that starting with a big dose right off the bat can be too much; if you can't handle the experience, it's less likely to be spiritual or comprehendible at all. Remember, there's no rush to get to a higher dose, and this isn't a competition to see who can handle the most. If you're curious about a higher-dose experience, work your way there by familiarizing your mind and your body with how psychedelics feel first. Especially if you don't have a lot of experience altering your consciousness (like with cannabis or other substances, such as MDMA), it's important to slowly work your way up to avoid overwhelming yourself.

MORE EXPERIENCED OR MODERATE DOSE?

So, you've tried about 1 gram and it was interesting, but you're looking to go deeper? Before you dive headfirst into a heroic dose, I would recommend experimenting with a moderate dose. Depending on the strength of the dried mushrooms, a moderate dose is in the ballpark of between 1.5 to 2.5 grams. The experience will definitely be stronger in this range, and it may be as high as you need to go. At a moderate dose, you'll be able to practice and hone in on your tripping navigation skills as well as get accustomed to the full-on tripping experience.

For many who use mushrooms somewhat frequently, this is considered a great social amount. With some psychedelic experience, this is the type of dose you can take with friends or loved ones to connect on a deeper level and to laugh together at all the absurdities of life. At this dose, experienced psychonauts could enjoy being outside in nature and taking a low-effort hike, especially after the mushrooms have peaked. However, for new mushroom users this will likely be a strong experience, so take it slow and don't push yourself to do too much if you're not up to it (literally, it can be hard to stand up).

However, one thing that's important to remember about low and moderate doses is they don't guarantee a pleasant or relaxing trip. In fact, many people find that low to moderate doses bring up a lot of negative feelings without "transcendence," which is more common at higher doses. In "Using Psychedelics Wisely," author and original psychedelic researcher of the 1960s Myron Stolaroff also makes this point but emphasizes the importance of working through these difficult emotions.

> *"Many do not like to use low doses because these [uncomfortable] feelings come to the surface. Rather than experience them, they use larger doses to transcend them. But these uncomfortable feelings are precisely what we must resolve to free ourselves from the Shadow, gain strength and energy, and function more comfortably and competently in the world. By using smaller amounts and being willing to focus our full attention on whatever feelings arise and breathe through them, we find that these feelings eventually dissolve, often with fresh insight and understanding of our personal dynamics. The release of such material permits an expansion of awareness and energy. If we work persistently to clear away repressed areas, we can enter the same sublime states that are available with larger doses— with an important additional gain. Having resolved our uncomfortable feelings, we are in a much better position to maintain a high state of clarity and functioning in day-to-day life."[87]*

I often find this to be the case; at doses above 3 grams, sometimes I "transcend" my problems and get this mystical feeling like I've got everything figured out and there's no need to doubt myself. However, unlike Stolaroff describes, at low and moderate doses, I can get stuck in negativity. It's still no reason to rush to a higher dose, yet, it's important to note because if you're having challenging experiences at low and moderate doses, it doesn't mean you should give up on mushrooms. Instead, be patient and gentle with yourself, and try to see what these challenging

87　Stolaroff, "Using Psychedelics Wisely."

experiences are trying to teach you. And when you're ready, you will hopefully be able to let go and have a different type of experience on a higher dose.

HIGH OR "HEROIC" DOSE

I would consider a high dose of psilocybin to be anywhere between 3 and 5 grams of dried mushrooms. Terence McKenna famously nicknamed a 5-gram journey the "heroic dose" because of its strong effects. That's because, at these higher doses, mystical or spiritual experiences are more likely, though obviously not guaranteed. What's also more likely at higher doses is the experience of ego loss and ego death, as well as the feeling that you've lost your mind and you're never getting it back. It can be a terrifying experience, and there is even the possibility of being traumatized by a high-dose trip you aren't prepared for,[88] which is why I emphasize that people slowly work their way up to a dose in this range.

Once you're familiar with how it feels to trip and you've developed some navigation skills like those I'll describe more in Chapter 9, you'll be better equipped to handle more intense high-dose experiences. You'll be better able to support yourself and remember somewhere in the back of your mind that you've taken a psychoactive substance and the feeling will eventually pass, whether it's terrifying or blissful. All in all, the important thing to remember is to start low and go slow, and never rush into a high dose experience without thoroughly preparing on lower dose trips first.

---

88   Conversation with Dr. Erica Zelfand, ND.

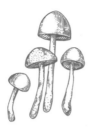

Chapter 8

WHAT TO EXPECT

WHAT DOES TRIPPING ON MUSHROOMS FEEL LIKE?

It's a simple question with a next-to-impossible answer. The psychedelic experience is famously ineffable, yet there are some common physical and mental sensations that I can describe. However, it's important to note that the effects of mushrooms are slightly different for everyone, and expectations have a large part in how psychedelics are experienced. While it's helpful to prepare yourself for the foreign feeling, I wouldn't get too bogged down in the details of how others experience mushrooms. Instead, simply trust and embrace the sensations as they come.

I know the mushrooms are starting to kick in when my body feels different; it starts with an almost tingling sensation, like butterflies in my stomach. Eventually, my body (especially my limbs) feels heavier, like it would take an incredible amount of energy to do a simple task. I can still get up and walk around if I have to, but because of this sensation, my balance is often a little off. Almost akin to being drunk, I don't walk in a straight line and move at a much slower pace than usual. I'll also weirdly yawn when the mushrooms have a strong hold on my system, even though tired is the last thing I'm feeling.

In addition, I can tell the mushrooms are starting to take effect when my eyes become more sensitive to light. I'll find myself squinting at a level of brightness that didn't bother me before. Usually around this time, my pupils dilate and stay quite large for the bulk of my trip. Then I'll look at things I see every day, like my own hands, and they seem a bit foreign and weird; I know that they're mine, but it's as if I've never seen them like this before. That's how the visuals begin for me; everything looks slightly different, even if I can't put my finger on how. Simple things can appear more beautiful than usual: the way sunlight hits a blade of grass can seem like poetry. Visuals can plateau here for some people depending on the dose, but there's also the possibility of a whole world of far-out visual sensations.

While the visual experience will be different for every individual, there are some common themes. When I first started using mushrooms, I knew I was in deep when everything seemed to breathe: the walls of my room, the floor, the ceiling—everything had a steady respiratory system. Things would sway and patterns would emerge, especially when I stared at certain textures and let my eyes rest. For example, anything wood, with its natural lines and grains, would dance around with liquid fluidity. Sometimes faces, patterns, and other geometric shapes in the wooden furniture or floorboards would "reveal" themselves to me. At higher doses, I've seen things melt, like my own face in the mirror, which also looks foreign even though I recognize it as mine. Others have told me of experiencing solid things as liquids, like the floor or a table, as well as other similarly weird changes in their everyday landscapes.

Despite the myths and urban legends, while your eyes are open, it's uncommon to hallucinate objects that aren't actually there. I ask Bill Richards about this and he agrees, that real hallucinations *can* happen, often coupled with loss of judgment and reality, but it's "extremely, extremely rare." He estimates that one participant in every 300 or so might experience "true" hallucinations where the tripper can't tell that what they're seeing isn't really there. What's more likely is a distortion of reality that you recognize as part of the psychedelic experience, like seeing geometric patterns. It's when your eyes are closed and you are relaxed that you can have "visions." "I like to use the term 'vivid mental imagery,'" Richards tells me, explaining when you close your eyes on mushrooms is when you'll see clear, sharply focused images that are much more easily remembered than a nocturnal dream.

Synesthesia is another visual sensation that people report. It's a perceptual phenomenon where one sense stimulates another. A small percentage of the population experiences this in everyday life, but under the influence of psilocybin, anyone can get a glimpse into the life of a "synesthete." A common type of synesthesia is experiencing sounds as colors, known as chromesthesia. While tripping, many experience this as "seeing" music, but there can be all types of synesthetic sensations.

Lastly, it's important to point out that the visual experience mushrooms produce can be drastically different for two people, even on the same dose of the same batch of fungi. While one person may be experiencing a lot of visuals, the other might not see any, but that doesn't mean they aren't tripping. If you're someone who doesn't experience a lot of visuals, don't beat yourself up over it because that can spiral into a negative headspace and definitely don't take another dose of mushrooms thinking they aren't working. Instead, embrace how the mushrooms do feel for you and be curious as to what they're trying to show or teach you. Closing your eyes and seeing where your thoughts take you can definitely help, both in terms of seeing visuals with your eyes closed or experiencing the mushrooms as more mind opening rather than eye opening.

While auditory hallucinations are practically unheard of with psilocybin, mushrooms can still distort your sense of hearing slightly. Especially if you're in a large, empty space prone to reverberation, mushrooms can amplify the echo, making it hard to hear the person who's talking to you. Others speak of the auditory distortion in terms of improving their hearing, that they tune in to sounds, like ants walking, that they would never be able to hear during a regular day.[89] Considering you experience all of your senses a bit differently on mushrooms, it's not totally surprising that they can have these auditory effects.

Because you also feel your body in a new way, certain things can feel more acute, like your posture or aches and pains. This can also contribute to the nausea that you may feel; it can be more a reaction to experiencing your body in a novel way than normal queasiness. However, mushrooms may upset your stomach,

89   Stamets, "1035: Joe Rogan Experience"

especially if you ate a lot before ingesting them or have a sensitive digestive system to begin with. There are a couple of things you can do to prevent and remedy this. Like we mentioned in Chapter 5 on preparing your set and setting, eating only a light, healthy meal a few hours before your trip can help prevent nausea. Many people with sensitive stomachs also recommend eating the mushrooms in the form of a tea (see the recipe in Chapter 5 for directions) to prevent nausea and throwing up. If you're feeling nauseous after the mushrooms have kicked in, try eating some kind of ginger product, like ginger ale or candy. Just focusing on your breathing and reminding yourself that it will pass can also help. If the nausea is the dominating sensation of your trip, you might want to try going to the bathroom and letting it come up if it has to. I wouldn't worry too much about not feeling the psychedelic effects if you do have to throw up—you're likely already tripping and the release will be a major relief.

How mushrooms feel in the mind is even harder to explain. Many describe the psychedelic experience in terms of expanding consciousness or softening the boundaries of the ego, giving more contact with the subconscious and less distinction between self and other. It also gives you a new perspective on things, whether that is yourself and your life, or the physical objects around you. You see and experience the world in a novel way, which is a big part of the allure. The expanded consciousness effect can lead to a lot of different emotional experiences. For instance, your thoughts can be very real and honest, helping you to realize things about yourself, your choices, and your struggles. This shift in perspective is the main reason why I, personally, use psychedelics occasionally. They help me step out of my everyday grind and see things with more clarity and with less baggage. I often realize things about my life or about life itself that can impact me greatly. The mushroom experience can be a catalyst for change for people because of this. People report quitting smoking, drinking, and other addictive or obsessive behaviors after a strong psychedelic experience, as well as leaving unhappy relationships, cutting meat and processed food from their diets, taking better care of the environment, or having less anxiety about things like death, change, and personal appearance, just to name a few.[90, 91, 92, 93]

Expanding your consciousness can also open the floodgates (quite literally) to sad emotions, past traumas, and tears. More so than other psychedelics, mushrooms make you emotional and can make you cry easily. This isn't necessarily a bad thing, often these painful emotions are pushed down for so long that when they bubble up on psilocybin it can feel cathartic, especially having a good cry over them. While the experience may be challenging, it may also be a sign that these are emotions that need to be dealt with, and you can continue to do so in more productive ways in your everyday life. This is part of the reason psilocybin can help with depression, PTSD, and anxiety, but proper integration is needed for the most positive effects. Yet, this is also why many who use mushrooms outside of official channels call it an emotional reset. They're able to put all their cards on the table and learn what needs to be dealt with after the effects of the mushrooms wear off.

90 Johnson, et al., "An Online Survey of Tobacco."

91 Garcia-Romeu, et al, "Cessation and Reduction in Alcohol Consumption."

92 Pisano, et al., "The Association of Psychedelic Use."

93 Lyons and Carhart-Harris, "Increased Nature Relatedness."

Mushrooms can also be really freeing for some people, especially at higher doses. It can be a feeling bursting with love, gratitude, and appreciation. There can also be a euphoric effect where it feels like you've transcended all of your problems, which can be a real source of strength for people. Through my research and interviews I found a common theme of realizations that different folks came to, that essentially, "Nothing matters." Although it sounds somewhat cynical or nihilistic, under the influence of mushrooms many people realize that all the little things that cause them so much stress and anxiety every day are actually quite trivial. This can help to give people strength during their non-tripping state—rather than existential dread—because they can stop themselves from getting worked up about little things by taking a breath, remembering it doesn't really matter in the big picture, and moving on.

Speaking of the grand scheme of things, because mushrooms can give you the sense of having an insider's view of how the world works, everyday objects and expectations can also seem absurd, silly, and even hysterically funny. In fact, I don't think I ever laugh as hard or as earnestly as when I'm on mushrooms. Sharing these silly insights and observations with your tripping partners can lead to uncontrollable giggles, which can be very therapeutic in itself. Plus, classic psychedelics can imbue such a sense of wonder and playfulness that it can feel like you're a kid again. It can also be a vulnerable feeling, but embracing it by acting goofy, playing imaginary games, or cuddling and sharing your feelings without restraint can be a wonderful experience.

A warped sense of time is also common. Time is another part of everyday life that can seem sort of funny or irrelevant while you're on psilocybin, and your sense of it will definitely be different. A four- to six-hour mushroom trip can feel a lot longer; part of why it's called a trip in the first place. Unless you're counting down the seconds for the mushrooms to wear off, this shouldn't really matter too much, although you might be shocked when you check the time. If you're not enjoying yourself, this warped sense of time can be your enemy, but instead of checking the clock obsessively, try asking yourself what's preventing you from having a good time and show compassion and curiosity for that feeling.

Another common tripping sensation is that of connectedness. It can be a feeling of strong connection to your tripping partners, to nature, or to the entire universe. It can also feel like there's less distinction between you and the rest of the world, that the boundaries of self and other are minimized. At higher doses this feeling becomes more common and can be part of a spiritual or mystical experience for some. When your ego recedes to this extent, it can feel like you are an integral part of nature, the universe, and the "divine plan," that you can talk to god, or even that you are a god. It can be a very powerful and positive experience, but there's a double edge to the "ego-loss coin." On the other side, it's possible to forget who and where you are, which can feel like going insane and that you're never coming back. At this point, you may be too far gone to remind yourself that this feeling shall pass and it is caused by a psychoactive substance you ingested, but these types of reminders can be very comforting, even if you don't fully believe or understand them in the moment. It's one of the reasons I suggest you work up to a high-dose experience, and it's also a good reason to enlist a guide or sitter for your first trip or a high-dose journey.

It's important to note that the intensity of the experience comes in waves. The most powerful part of the trip, often called the "peak," comes around two to three hours after eating mushrooms. But you're still tripping after your peak for another two to four hours, and this is where the waves become most apparent. Four or five hours after you've eaten the mushrooms, it may feel like they've worn off (especially compared to the intensity of your peak), but then another wave of the psychedelic experience could hit you. That's why it's important to set aside the whole day for your trip because a new wave of insight, tears, or visuals could surprise you. Moreover, even after the waves subside, you will still be in an emotionally sensitive place into the next day or two.

Finally, the days following your trip are also something to prepare for. Many people report feeling an "afterglow"; this can mean different things for different people. For me, especially the day immediately following a trip, it's like having a foot in both worlds, the mushroom one and the "real" one. If I had a challenging trip, my afterglow can look more like vulnerability and a rawness of emotions. I can break down into tears much more easily than usual, but sometimes that's exactly the medicine I need. On the other hand, if I'm waking up after a powerfully positive trip, I can feel great and free of anxiety the next day. As in all things with magic mushrooms, afterglow is a very subjective experience. Either way, I personally prefer to be home that day to sit with those emotions—whether they're good or bad—they're usually important to my whole experience, so I like to digest and ponder them.

Chapter 9

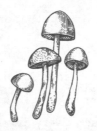

HOW TO NAVIGATE THE SPACE

Trust. Let Go. Be Open.

—Bill Richards, *Sacred Knowledge*

Navigating the psychedelic experience isn't always intuitive and takes some practice and skills. Getting comfortable in the space can be the hardest part, as it is so dramatically different from everyday life that it can be overwhelming or frightening. But according to researchers, the most important thing you can do is to approach the experience with an accepting attitude and open mind.[94] Similarly, while you're actually under the influence of a psychedelic, the most important navigation skill is to relax. It sounds simple—too easy, even—but relinquishing your control to the substance, to not resist its powers and just let go and see where it takes you, can be challenging. In fact, you might not

94   Watts and Luoma, "The Use of the Psychological Flexibility."

even realize you're resisting the effects, which is another reason why I recommend tripping on lower doses first. It will give you time to get used to the physical and mental sensations and learn how to "let go" before moving on to more intense experiences.

In one of the first trip manuals, *The Psychedelic Experience*, published in 1964, the main recommendation for tripping successfully still holds true: "Whenever in doubt, turn off your mind, relax, float downstream." In fact, every psychedelic expert who has written on the subject has given this same advice in their own words. Rick Strassman, author of *DMT: The Spirit Molecule*, and the first scientist to resume psychedelic research since prohibition, advises something very similar: "It is only through letting go that we find ourselves making the most progress… this surrender is the crux of a successful journey."[95]

Similarly, in *The Psychedelic Explorers' Guide*, James Fadiman gives more specifics on how to surrender: "Observe what is going on inside your mind and body, but do not try to control the flow of images and sensations. Allow your mind to take its natural course; relax and observe as your thoughts unfold without any effort. Affirm that all experiences are welcome."[96] Fadiman's advice is crucial because it not only recommends relaxing and surrendering to the experience, but it reminds us that we shouldn't try to control every thought, and just accept and welcome them as they come. However, while you're tripping, this can be difficult because your mind will constantly try to rationalize everything.

---

95 Strassman, R., Wojtowicz, S., Luna, L.E., and Frecka, E. *Inner Paths to Outer Space: Journeys to Alien Worlds through Psychedelics and Other Spiritual Technologies.*
96 Fadiman, *The Psychedelic Explorers' Guide.*

This happened to me very recently on a high-dose trip. I was having profound realizations about the nature of my life and personality, but even with 4 grams of mushrooms in my system, my mind was still trying to figure out and rationalize all of my insights. I had to keep reminding myself that midtrip wasn't the time to figure out all the details. Even though I had realized all these things about myself, I didn't need to make a plan that instant about how I was going to change all these aspects of my life. Yet my brain still struggled, because when I'm sober, I make plans to fix problems almost immediately; it's how I'm wired. But while tripping, I knew that I could go deeper if I just saw these problems from a new angle, made a mental note of them, and showed them curiosity and forgiveness rather than solutions or explanations. Then I could let the mushrooms show me more rather than get stuck trying to figure it all out. That helped me to stop resisting and trying to control the mushroom experience. And I did go deeper. I reached a blissful all-knowing place where everything was figured out and there was nothing to be worried about. I laughed out loud at all of my "silly human problems" and had my first mystical experience on psychedelics.

This is where having a practice of meditation in your daily life can help you navigate the psychedelic space, because in meditation you learn how to relax your mind and let thoughts come and go without engaging them. Our minds naturally rationalize and judge everything around us—it's a safety mechanism to keep us alive, so it's completely unnatural for us to stop doing so, whether we're on mushrooms or not. While I'm terrible at meditating, I was still practicing before my latest psychedelic experience, and I was able to use that developing skill to stop resisting and rationalizing everything and, instead, relax and go deeper.

So if you find yourself being overly critical of your thoughts while you're tripping, try taking a deep breath, closing your eyes, and simply focus on your breathing. In fact, remembering to breathe and doing so deeply and mindfully is the other crucial navigation skill. It can also help to have music playing. Try focusing on the music while breathing and relaxing your mind. This might also be a good time to repeat a mantra. For me, thinking: "Teach me, I'm listening" helped me to stop rationalizing, judging, and planning everything, and just be in the moment. But sticking to the classic: "Trust, let go, be open," should do the trick, too. Before the trip begins, choose a mantra that encourages you to be calm, present, and accepting of the experience, no matter what it is.

In his tripping manual, *Preparation for the Journey,* Strassman recommends people first lay a strong foundation of "inner work skills," like psychotherapy or meditation, long before experimenting with psychedelics. Strassman writes: "These skills make it easier to remain focused when confronted with the unexpected. In addition, effective psychotherapy or spiritual practice will have made us familiar with the skeletons in our closets and will have better equipped us to contend with them if and when they emerge. Thus, not only do we clearly perceive what is garnering our attention, but also we subsequently open up and drop our resistances to it."

Yet, in an essay called "Using Psychedelics Wisely," Myron Stolaroff points out that while psychedelics can help us reveal the unconscious, we can't forget that our minds have repressed those thoughts and memories for a reason. "We may not welcome the appearance of repressed, painful feelings, or of evidence that our values and lifestyles might be considerably improved. Nor is it always easy to accept the spaciousness of our being, our immense potential, and the responsibility that these entail," writes Stolaroff. Later in the same essay he warns that if you are taking psychedelics for pleasure, you might find yourself overwhelmed "by the eruption of repressed unconscious material without knowing how to deal with it."

That's one of the reasons it has been argued that being in a stable place and having a firm sense of who you are and your purpose in this world will help you have a meaningful trip. Richards writes a similar sentiment in his essay, "Navigation within Consciousness"—"Those who have pursued dynamically oriented psychotherapy or self-exploration know the paradox that one must have a reasonably strong ego, a developed sense of self, before one can feel sufficiently safe in the world to choose unconditionally to trust so-called deeper or higher dimensions of being within consciousness."[97] When I ask Dr. Erica Zelfand, ND and psychedelic integration provider, about this, she puts it in simple terms: "You can't launch into outer space without good ground control." Meaning, you need to be able to regulate yourself and your emotions, and really be able to resource yourself internally, before jumping into such an altered state of consciousness.

But how do you know if you have "good ground control"? We'll get more into who should take extra precautions with psychedelics and why in Chapter 14, but an important navigation skill is knowing when it's the wrong time to trip. Thoughtfully consider

97   Richards, "Navigation Within Consciousness."

where you're at emotionally before planning a psychedelic experience. These substances are not an escape from your life or your problems but rather quite the opposite. A trip fosters a deeper look at yourself from a new angle, so being prepared to have painful feelings bubble up is important. You might realize things you haven't fully dealt with emotionally, like trauma or grief, and it can be challenging but also rewarding. Consider whether you're in the right emotional state to tackle these issues, and if not, there's no harm in waiting until you are.

Tripping can get scary, even if you do have a strong sense of who you are and are in a stable place in your life. Richards has also written "Flight Instructions" for researchers who guide participants through psychedelic experiences in clinical trials. In it, he recommends a bunch of phrases for guides to tell trippers to help them release their control to the substance and go deeper, such as:

- "Trust. Let go. Be open."
- "Trust the trajectory, follow your path."
- "If you feel like you're dying, melting, dissolving, exploding, going crazy, etc.—go ahead, embrace it."[98]

You can try telling yourself one or more of these phrases as a mantra, or even write one down on a piece of paper and stick it on the ceiling above your bed before ingesting a psychedelic. Richards also has advice for when and if the trip gets dark or if participants feel fear or anxiety; he advises guides to encourage trippers to face their fear. "Look the monster in the eye and move toward it... Dig in your heels; ask, 'What are you doing in my mind?' Or, 'What can I learn from you?'" Through his

---

98   Richards, "Flight Instructions."

experience guiding hundreds through psychedelic journeys, he's learned that when you encourage people to literally face their demons, a transformation can occur. The symbolic monster could turn into whatever in their subconscious is troubling them, whether it is an abusive parent, the fear of failure, or unresolved grief or guilt. He writes this transformation is usually followed by catharsis and understanding. "What is so important here is the discovery that the monster has meaning and in itself is an invitation to enhanced psychological health and spiritual maturation. Its purpose is not to torment, but to teach," Richards writes in *Sacred Knowledge*.

It's important to note here that the strength to face your demons while tripping may come from having a strong support system such as in clinical trials with psilocybin, and doing this on your own at home might not be as successful or easy. But as many experienced psychonauts well know, bad trips only get worse when you run from the monster, and catharsis comes from facing your "shadow." We'll get more into how to deal with and avoid bad trips in the next chapter, but if you plan on doing mushrooms for healing, it's probably in your best interest to enlist a supportive sitter at the very least, and seriously consider getting a professional guide or shaman, going to a retreat, or applying for a clinical trial, as mentioned in Chapter 6.

Another common way a mushroom trip can turn sour is if you get stuck in what many psychonauts refer to as a "negative thought loop." This is when you have overly negative thoughts, usually fueled by anxiety, that repeat or spiral into more anxious thinking. However, people who regularly use mushrooms at home have developed their own techniques to curb these negative loops. Basically, anything to distract yourself can help, which is why preparing some activities and supplies beforehand is a great thing to do. Like I mentioned in Chapter 5, having things like art supplies, coloring books, nature books or documentaries, fruit, or musical instruments can help get you out of a negative headspace. Changing the music or the scenery can also help, as can getting up and moving your body through dance, yoga, or just walking around. For this same reason, some people find having an altar to look at or a small rock or crystal to hold can help to keep them grounded or to refocus their attention. In general, it's important not to beat yourself up or push yourself in any way. When you've eaten mushrooms, you're in a very sensitive place, so being gentle and forgiving with yourself goes a long way.

Navigation Skills Summary:

- Be open and accepting to all experiences as they come.
- Relax and let your thoughts flow without trying to control them.
- Breathe deeply and mindfully.

Chapter 10

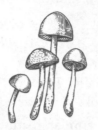

CHALLENGING TRIPS AND INTRODUCTION TO THE SHADOW

There's a saying in the psychedelic community that there's no such thing as a "bad trip," only challenging experiences. While I would agree to an extent that challenging trips can provide a great deal of healing or teach us the most about ourselves—I still think there's a distinction between a bad and a challenging trip. To me, a bad trip is one that wasn't prepared and planned for sufficiently, and so the set and setting are all wrong, and the whole experience is overwhelming, chaotic, and unnecessarily stressful. These "bad trip" experiences are common in recreational use, especially in younger and inexperienced folks, and often, not much is learned. On the other hand, a challenging trip is a journey that is well prepared for, but still ends up being difficult emotionally and sometimes physically. However, with the proper navigation skills, integration tools, and, often, the presence of a guide or sitter, challenging trips can be extremely rewarding experiences for personal growth.

James W. Jesso, host of the podcast *Adventures Through the Mind* and author of a few books on psychedelics, including *The True Light of Darkness*, makes a similar distinction. He defines a bad trip as "becoming overwhelmed by an anxiety resulted from the resistance of an altered state—i.e., wishing we were not high anymore or wishing the experience was different."[99] Jesso distinguishes this from a "hard trip," which he writes, "is when we are presented with the darker aspects of the self, the *shadow*. But instead of resisting the discomfort of that encounter, we embrace it, we *surrender* to it. It is these trips that hold the most potential for personal growth. And learning how to surrender into the honesty of emotional experience, especially if it is challenging, enables this growth most effectively."

If you recall in Chapter 9 on navigating the space, we high-lighted the fact that "letting go" and "relinquishing your control" to the psychedelic experience is paramount. You may still have a challenging experience, but resistance will only make it worse. On the other hand, acceptance can lead to true insight, and possibly, transcendence or catharsis on the other side. However, letting go will be impossible in a chaotic environment or if you are unprepared emotionally. Because you'll lack the ability to trust in your surroundings or yourself, you may find that you're grasping for straws of control, which can lead to more extreme

---

99   Jesso, *The True Light of Darkness*.

paranoia, confusion, and other unpleasant experiences, such as psychosomatic physical symptoms.

Challenging trips can take a lot of different forms, so it's important to prepare yourself. For instance, your visual experience can get quite dark; instead of things seeming otherworldly in their beauty, they can seem eerie and wrong somehow, which is likely to induce anxiety. In fact, James Giordano reminds me that a common reason people get anxiety during their first few trips is that the tripping sensation contrasts so much with their memory of reality, and that can be frightening. Whether it's how they experience their own minds, bodies, or physical surroundings, it's the change that scares people and causes them to resist. He says this is another reason having a guide or sitter could be helpful to psychedelic-naïve folks, to help talk them through disconcerting experiences.

It's also possible to relive painful memories, especially traumas. According to Stanislav Grof in his quintessential manual for psychedelic guides, *LSD Psychotherapy*, some participants can become convinced that they are dying and may even have physical symptoms to accompany this fear such as "seizure-like motor activity, projectile vomiting, profuse sweating, and fast thread-like pulse."[100] However, he assures guides that these are psychosomatic symptoms, not chemical reactions to the psychedelic, and the "total surrender to it is always followed by feelings of liberation, whereas struggle against it prolongs the suffering." Grof also points out two other important challenging trip experiences: the fear that the psychedelic experience will never end, and its related horror, that "permanent insanity is imminent." However, he explains that these are both reactions

100   Grof, *LSD Psychotherapy*.

rooted in the fear of losing control, and at this point you can guess the solution: letting go.

Yet, without a guide or sitter that you trust, letting go to these frightening experiences can be next to impossible, even if you're in a calm and safe environment. Edward, a 62-year-old man I interviewed for this book (name changed for privacy), told me of a harrowing experience he had taking 3 grams of psilocybin alone at home to deal with an early childhood trauma. Although he believes he was releasing his control to the experience and "just allowing it to happen," as he had read about previous to the journey, he was still overwhelmed by the trip. "My feelings were tumbling out of me," he tells me over the phone. "I was in complete anguish." He describes the experience as one of terror where his whole life was falling apart and he got stuck in a "deep flashback state." However, he laments, he never experienced "ego death" or transcended his traumas like the literature on psychedelics can promise. He realized he couldn't do this difficult healing work on his own and plans to enlist the help of a professional guide before embarking on his next psilocybin journey.

INTRODUCTION TO THE SHADOW

According to Grof and many other psychologists, psychedelics can "lower the threshold of your conscious," allowing more access to unconscious material. In a therapeutic setting, this is ideal, but when doing mushrooms on your own, you could be left to confront your shadow. The shadow is a concept in

Jungian psychology that is basically the negative side to your personality; the "sum of all those unpleasant qualities we like to hide."[101] Although Jung disapproved of psychedelic therapy in the 1950s,[102] psychedelic therapists have adapted many of his ideas to explain the experience, especially its healing properties. For instance, Jungian archetypes can be used to translate the images and visions we see during psychedelic journeys. His concept of the shadow is crucial when trying to understand the underlying benefit of challenging trips.

Ann Shulgin, matriarch of the psychedelic community, therapist, and coauthor of the classic psychedelic books *PiHKAL: A Chemical Love Story* and *TiHKAL: The Continuation* along with her late husband, renowned psychedelic chemist Alexander "Sasha" Shulgin, has written and spoken extensively on the topic of the shadow in psychedelic experiences. First of all, she makes it clear that the shadow isn't inherently bad or evil. Instead, it is what has been repressed since childhood. "Whatever has been forbidden and treated with contempt by the authority figures surrounding the child. It is those aspects of the person which he has come to think of as unacceptable, awful, terrible, unlovable, and even dangerous," Shulgin says of the shadow during a speech in 2002.[103] She explains that the more we repress our shadow qualities, the stronger they'll become, and we can begin to project these unwanted aspects of ourselves onto others. That's when our shadow can become destructive, because without realizing it, these projections damage personal and professional relationships.

---

101   Jung, *The Collected Works of C. G. Jung. Vol 7.*

102   Hill, *Confrontation with the Unconscious.*

103   Shulgin, "Psychedelic Psychotherapy and the Shadow."

But that's where psychedelics come in. Using psychedelics in a therapeutic setting, we can finally confront our shadow and bring it into the light. If done so with the proper support, we can show our shadow compassion—forgiveness even—and it can stop having so much power over us. "What happens... if we manage to bring it up to the light? It transforms; it changes," says Shulgin. "It's still there, but no longer as a monster. When you allow yourself to acknowledge, without fear and without hatred... you can allow yourself to have those darker thoughts and feelings, along with the more lovable and admirable ones. You become free."

Shulgin's ideas come from Jung's own theories. He wrote a similar sentiment in *Two Essays in Analytical Psychology*: "If people can be educated to see the shadow-side of their nature clearly, it may be hoped that they will also learn to understand and love their fellow men better. A little less hypocrisy and a little more self-knowledge can only have good results in respect for our neighbor; for we are all too prone to transfer to our fellows the injustices and violence we inflict upon our own natures."

It sounds great: By confronting your shadow on mushrooms you can become a better person! The only problem is, having the courage to face your personalized worst fears and release to it— to accept it without anxiety, shame, or resistance—is tough. It's another instance where having a guide, sitter, or ongoing practice of inner-work skills like meditation can be really beneficial. Like in Edward's case, sometimes you need that extra support or you can get stuck in the negativity without any transformation.

At the same time, in my personal experience, psilocybin can make me very forgiving and compassionate in general, and so when I've been confronted with some of my shadow qualities while tripping, I've been able to recognize them and show them love and forgiveness rather than the embarrassment and self-hatred they cause me—often unknowingly—in everyday life. Although not everyone gets to this self-love place as easily on mushrooms, I have found that it is a common experience when you stop fighting or denying ugly thoughts or negative realizations, and instead, accept them.

For example, recently on a medium-dose trip of 2.5 grams, I saw how selfish and demanding I can be in my relationship with my partner. It shamed me greatly, and tears came rolling down my cheeks at an unstoppable rate. But although it was challenging, my experience wasn't negative. I also saw how much my partner loves me and all that he does for me. It brought happy tears to my eyes because I was so grateful to have him in my life. The key is, I accepted it; I didn't disagree with this realization or try to fight it. But instead, I let this shadow quality of mine come into the light and started thinking of ways to change. It gave me great hope and an ecstatic, happy feeling knowing that I can choose to act in another way. This is where integration plays a big part. Now that I had this confrontation with my shadow, I can actively do things in my relationship to continue to confront my selfishness and not let it take over and ultimately destroy our connection. For me personally, my integration involves actively taking a bigger role in household chores like sweeping, making dinner, and walking the dogs. I didn't get rid of my shadow (I'm still selfish sometimes, but who isn't?), but now that I know sometimes I can be *too* selfish, I can step back and make adjustments to my behavior.

WAYS TO AVOID BAD TRIPS

Avoiding unnecessarily bad trips really comes down to adequate preparation. Like we've discussed in previous chapters, it's of critical importance to plan a comfortable, secure, and familiar setting. You need to be able to put 100 percent of your trust in not only your physical environment, but also the people you are with. Whether you're tripping with friends or loved ones, or you've enlisted a guide or sitter to keep you safe, you need to be able to trust them unconditionally to avoid a needlessly hard trip. Because your environment can have such a dramatic impact on your experience, I would highly recommend that you avoid using mushrooms in public situations, whether that be a music festival, city park, or amazing art exhibit. Sometimes these experiences can be enhanced safely by microdosing, which we'll discuss in more depth in Chapter 13, but for a dose higher than 0.5 grams, and especially for your first time, tripping in a private, secure location is the easiest way to avoid a bad experience.

But remember, setting is only half of the expression; you also need to be in the right set—aka mood or headspace—to avoid a bad trip. Like we discussed in Chapter 5, knowing when it's the wrong time to trip is critical, as is preparing yourself mentally and emotionally.

As noted above, the correct dose is also paramount to avoiding a bad trip. Like was discussed in Chapter 7, start with a small dose for your first psilocybin experience (or your first experience in a while) and work your way up to a higher-dose journey in subsequent trips. Learn the lay of the land before exceeding around 2 grams of dried mushrooms in order to prevent any resistance or anxiety. While all your trips will be somewhat different, having experience and practicing navigation skills will help you be more prepared for encountering challenging experiences on higher-dose journeys, and hopefully accepting or even transcending them.

WAYS TO DEAL WITH CHALLENGING TRIPS

Tripping can get challenging even if you plan the perfect, most tranquil set and setting and are with people you absolutely trust and adore or are doing so with an amazing facilitator. In guided psilocybin sessions, if you experience fear or are trying to control the situation too much, your guide should be knowledgeable enough to read your body language, facial expression, or breathing pattern and support you. This could come in the form of a reassuring touch, like hand-holding, offering you a blanket, or encouraging phrases to help you relax and face your demons. Remember how the number-one tripping navigation skill was letting go? Well, the main way to deal with a challenging trip is the same: You need to stop fighting and trying to control or end the situation and accept it, even offer it curiosity and compassion. "As with the nocturnal nightmares most of us can recall, when one runs away from psychological conflicts the threatening specter grows bigger and one feels weaker, smaller, and increasingly anxious, often awakening in a cold sweat," writes Richards in *Sacred Knowledge*. "When the frightening image is courageously approached and confronted, one grows stronger and insights awaken." Again, this confrontation is easier to do with a guide or experienced sitter, but the acceptance and resolution of a challenging trip can be a great source of personal growth.

I realize, however, that many of you will not be taking mushrooms in the presence of a guide or even a sitter, and some of you will not be doing them for "healing" either, so is there anything you can do to deal with challenging trips at home? Of course! If you're having a difficult experience, changing the scenery is one of the easiest ways to switch things up and transition from a super-negative headspace. Getting up to sit in another room, or going from inside to outside or vice versa, can do wonders for easing your experience. If you live in a small apartment and this isn't an option, don't leave home to try and sort things out. It will likely make you feel more anxious or overwhelmed. Instead, try sitting on a different piece of furniture or lying on the floor instead of the couch.

Changing the music is another easy thing you can do to lighten the mood when tripping gets tough. Music can have a profound effect on your state of mind while under the influence of psychedelics, and changing it can feel like you've entered a totally new space, and hopefully a lighter and more manageable one. If things get really hard and you can't seem to see it through or let go on your own, try moving on to one of the activities you planned. Remember in Chapter 5 we recommended downloading some nature documentaries to watch if things got tough, or taking some inspiring art or nature books from the library beforehand to look at? Well, this is the time to get those things out! Looking at fresh-cut flowers or other houseplants can also help, as can going outside for a nature walk if you have a yard or if you've rented a cabin. If you've made an altar, this would be a good time to visit it to refocus and re-center yourself. Other activities like dance, making art or music, or physical ways to release energy like shaking your limbs, singing, or even screaming could help. Other distractions like pretty lights, pieces of art, soft fabrics, or other interesting textures could also be just the thing to get you out of a challenging place.

While you might not get the most healing out of distracting yourself, sometimes doing that deep inner work can be too difficult on your own, and it's okay to find other ways to cope and relax. Don't force yourself to go inward and sit with your feelings if you can't release yourself to them. But if you think you can, try focusing on your breathing to stop fighting the experience and ask yourself or your shadow: Why are you here? What can I learn from you? It's important to approach your feelings with openness, acceptance, and curiosity rather than embarrassment, shame, or resistance. Taking deep breaths and holding on to a little crystal or rock can help to keep you grounded while you release yourself to the experience. Speaking of being grounded, many experts recommend taking off your shoes and touching your bare feet to the floor or earth. Plus, don't forget that breathing through difficult emotions or sensations is one of the most important navigation skills and ways to re-center yourself during a challenging experience!

If you're with friends or loved ones while your trip is getting particularly challenging, tell them. You don't have to go into too much detail or try to figure everything out through talking to them, but a supportive touch like holding hands, or hugging or cuddling if you're close, can really help. So reach out to your friends and cuddle under a blanket if your inner experience is getting too tough to manage on your own; they'll probably be glad you did!

Sometimes experiences are challenging due to physical sensations, like pain, nausea, or twitches and sudden jerky movements. Again, don't fight these feelings, just let them play themselves out—without hurting yourself or anyone else—and you'll likely feel much better afterward. In the case of nausea, throwing up can really help, not just with the nausea but with release in general, so don't fight it. Instead, try to get yourself to the bathroom and let it come up.

For those with a meditation practice, it can really help in these situations as well. Jesso describes how meditating for just 10 to 15 minutes when a psilocybin trip got really difficult helped to re-center him. "Finding a small corner to sit in, I placed my hands on my heart and began to meditate. This was what I had needed the whole time, an opportunity to just sit and be present with myself. I breathed with intention, bringing forgiveness and compassion on my inhalations, releasing tension and stress in my exhalations. I didn't avoid my hard feelings anymore, but sat with them while cultivating a sense of worthiness and self-love. It must have been at least 15 minutes before the guys emerged from huntergathering our dinner out from the chaos that is an affluent Canadian food supply chain store during rush hour. And by that time, I was feeling much better."[104]

Whatever it takes to get you grounded, re-centered, and calm is going to be the best way to dig yourself out of a challenging trip.

---

104   Jesso, *The True Light of Darkness.*

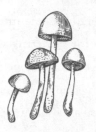

Chapter 11

INTEGRATION

*It's not the substance but
how we employ the substance in service
to an ethic that gets results.*

—Bett Williams, *The Wild Kindness*

Integration is arguably one of the most misunderstood concepts in psychedelics. In fact, as research for this book, when I interviewed people who occasionally use mushrooms and asked them what integration meant to them, many said "nothing." But it's actually not a very complicated idea. Integration is making sense of a psychedelic experience, mining it for lessons or insights, and then applying those teachings to your everyday life. And because everyone's psychedelic experience is unique to them, integration also looks very different for each individual.

Integration is a crucial step to using mushrooms and other psychedelics for personal growth. Simply taking mushrooms alone doesn't guarantee any kind of long-term personality change, but as the psychedelic community likes to say, it can be a catalyst for growth—for realizing what kind of changes you need to make in order to become a better, more fulfilled person. "It's not about integrating the experience," says Erica Zelfand, who provides integration as a naturopathic doctor, "it's about integrating the human."

Zelfand has a great analogy that she shared with me over the phone. She compared integration to the story of the Ten Commandments, when Moses received two inscribed tablets at the top of Mount Sinai—his mystical experience. "But he can't stay on the mountain forever," says Zelfand, "that's not where life is." He has to take the tablets and his newfound wisdom back to his community, she explains. They examine them and think, "How can we live in alignment with this new wisdom? How can we use this wisdom to level up?" And that's exactly what psychedelic integration is. Taking the newfound knowledge, insights, or revelations you have during psychedelic experiences and bringing them down the mountain, unpacking them, and deciding how to use that information and how it fits into your life. "And it doesn't have to all necessarily make sense in a linear fashion," points out Zelfand. "But, how can I use this to be a more authentic, wonderful version of myself? How can I use this to grow in a way beyond having a fun or beautiful night where I tripped out?"

When I ask Elizabeth Nielson, who not only provides psychedelic integration in private practice and clinical trials but also trains clinicians on integration, the same question, "What is psychedelic integration?" she has a similar answer. "I think of it as finding the insights that one has had during a psychedelic experience—or any experience really—and moving it to the larger canvas of one's life." She explains how psychedelic experiences can be really intense; people can access new knowledge or new ways of thinking of things. "But those things may be sort of ephemeral, fragile, or even easily discounted depending on the context. And so integration is really taking those insights and investing in them. Figuring out which ones are valuable and how they're valuable. And then remembering them, practicing them, making longer term changes based on them in a way that should be positive and promoting longer term health and wellness."

Some lessons will be clear. For example, going into a recent trip, I was feeling isolated and disconnected, wondering why more people didn't reach out to me for my birthday. But then on mushrooms, I saw very clearly it wasn't that my friends and family didn't love me, or some kind of innate inability on my part to develop close connections. Instead, it's that I put up boundaries that people are respecting. I also saw that the solution was easy, that I was making a choice to put up those boundaries, but I could choose differently by telling people how I feel and letting them in by reaching out more. In fact, I saw that everything in life was a choice, and I've been making choices that make me unhappy and anxious.

These lessons were crystal clear during my trip, but integrating them, acting on them, and making changes is much harder and less straightforward. Integration is a journey, and I'm still very much on it months after this particular voyage. A big part of my process has been trying to call my friends and family more, and to reach out to other family members who aren't on my weekly call rotation. At first it was also trying to make more new friends, and I was pushing myself to go out more to parties and events in town to meet new people. But after some unsuccessful attempts to meet up with new acquaintances, yet some great weekends with reliable old friends, I realized to enact the lessons from my trip, I really needed to invest more in the relationships I already had. Integrating my other lesson, that everything is a choice—including my sometimes-crippling social anxiety—is harder. I can't flip a switch and become confident, but I can choose—or try through some mindfulness—to be less hard on myself and engage in less negative self-talk that fuels my anxiety and insecurity. Is it working? Well, like Bill Richards told me when I asked him about integration, "It's a lifelong process." So I'll have to get back to you.

Ros Watts gave me a similar example of what integration could look like from a follow-up session she had just conducted with a clinical trial participant before I called her. She explained that the person she had been working with was a perfectionist, so for her, a big part of her integration is learning to embrace her imperfections and giving herself a break when she doesn't do things right. "It's just a very subtle thing that will hopefully percolate her whole life," says Watts. "It's not going to be one big thing she does or doesn't do. It's going to be a subtle layer of the way she talks to herself and the way she is with herself."

All the experts I spoke with for this chapter agreed that putting the lessons you learn during a psychedelic experience into practice is the hardest part of this whole process of using psychedelics for personal growth and lasting change. Nielson explains that it's especially hard if we're talking about changes in behavior, habits, and interpersonal relationships. It's one thing if you realize you need to spend more time out in nature, but quite another to see that you have to change your whole way of talking to yourself or to others. Yet at the same time, choosing the lessons with value and how to incorporate them into your life can also be tricky. Zelfand points out that you can have a vision of yourself quitting your job and money flying at you, but are you going to drop out of your life, move off the grid, and expect it all to work out? Maybe a more productive way to integrate that lesson would be to look at changing careers so you have to hustle for money less or moving into a smaller apartment or cheaper city to reduce your cost of living. But figuring that out will take some reflection.

Interestingly, in clinical trials with psilocybin, guides advise participants not to make any major life changes immediately—like leaving a spouse or quitting a job—following a "dosing session," but rather to give the experience a little time to digest first. Basically, take a few weeks to reflect on your lessons before deciding the best way to act on them. Nielson also points out that, just like in psychedelic therapy where participants are told to trust their "inner healing intelligence," the same concept applies to integration. "It's sort of a fancier term for intuition," Nielson says. "People really benefit when they are empowered to follow their own intuition and find things that work for them." She explains that a big part of her work as an integration therapist in private practice is helping people trust themselves. "Oftentimes people don't fully trust themselves," she says. "So it's really important that I trust them and model that trust in them and provide a space that's safe and open for them to explore the things that they think are right for themselves." And so after some serious reflection on your psychedelic experience, trust your gut on how to proceed with your integration.

INTEGRATION TECHNIQUES

It isn't always simple to find the lessons from your trip. You need to figure them out before you can begin to act on them. That's where integration techniques come in. Many of the practices below can help you reflect on your trip and figure out how it fits in with the rest of your life. There's no formula to integration, as Nielson also points out to me, and it'll be unique to the individual and their psychedelic experience. Again, it's important to listen to your instinct—or inner healing wisdom—to see which of these activities speak to you. It's not necessary to start a new practice, like meditation or yoga, to integrate, but if it resonates with you, give it a try!

JOURNALING AND OTHER FORMS OF SELF-EXPRESSION AND REFLECTION

The most popular and highly encouraged technique for integration is journaling. Starting a journal before your trip and continuing to use it in the days and weeks afterward to reflect on your experience is one of the best ways to help you find meaning. What's more, going back and reading your journal entries weeks, months, or even years later can also help you make sense of a journey and give you an opportunity to reflect on your growth.

There's no formula to journaling, but I would recommend starting before your trip by writing about your intentions, expectations, fears, and hopes. You can bring your journal along for your psychedelic experience to capture any realizations or insights in the moment, but this becomes harder as doses get higher, so don't feel it's necessary to write during your trip. But a great time to write about the actual journey, its sensations, visions, and insights, will be once the mushrooms have worn off. If you're not too tired, start capturing how you're feeling and the visceral sensations from your experience the same day as your trip. In the days and weeks following your experience, continue to journal, reflecting on that experience, what it meant to you, how you're feeling now in the aftermath, and any other feelings or insights you may come to. Often just by writing these things out, new lessons and realizations become clear, and reading them later can really help to reinforce or reinterpret them.

Journaling doesn't have to be only written content either. In fact, integration is more about reflection and self-expression than it is recording every detail of your trip. If creating art or music is more your speed, then these can be great ways to begin integrating and mining your trip for lessons. Especially if your experience is hard to put into words or to make much sense of, try drawing, painting, singing, or making other forms of art or music to begin to work through it. "One of the values in this is that it can help you physically move the experience from being something that's contained in one's mind to something that is in another position in relation to you that you can then reflect on," says Nielson. "If you make a drawing that represents a piece of your experience, you can then look at that drawing and observe things about it that you might not notice if it's still something that you're picturing in your mind. And you may notice further details about it that you hadn't before." She says that drawing or writing about your experience isn't required for integration, but they are useful tools to help you gain perspective.

COMMUNITY

Community can mean a lot of things. But one helpful way to unpack and integrate your experience is by talking about it with people. If you have friends, family, or other loved ones with psychedelic experience, that's a great place to start. But because these substances are still criminalized and highly stigmatized, it's common not to have anyone in your circle to discuss these experiences with, without sounding a bit like you fell off your rocker. That's where integration groups come in. Popping up all over the US, especially in major cities like New York, San Francisco, and Los Angeles, public integration meetups are now an option. They're often called names like "integration circle" or "psychedelic society," and can be found online on sites like Eventbrite and Meetup. Typically, they are held in public spaces where people can come for free to listen and share with a group of open-minded people with similar experiences.

"It's lovely for connecting people and getting a community together," says Ros Watts who, in addition to working on psychedelic clinical trials, hosts a public integration group in London. She explains that after a psychedelic experience, it's typical for people to realize there are other ways to live their lives and manage their pain. "It's a new way of exploring yourself by choosing to go into painful places. Because every time you have a psychedelic experience, you're opening up to the possibility that you might have a really, really very difficult time," she says. And so, having a group of like-minded people to talk about these things with is helpful because "it feels like a group of people that have all made this commitment to really explore their inner worlds. So it's really nice for them to meet other people that are doing the same thing," says Watts.

Elizabeth Nielson has also hosted a public integration group in New York City, and although she agrees that having community to integrate with can be very helpful for some people, she explains there can also be some drawbacks. For one, she says that because these meetings are public, they don't have the same doctor-patient confidentiality that seeing a private, licensed integration therapist does. And so, there's a risk that someone could inadvertently reveal your psychedelic use to the public or to a coworker, which could get some people in serious trouble. She also says that sometimes public groups attract people who may not be in a safe, stable emotional place and the way they share things with others could be upsetting or triggering to some. "Sometimes they're fabulously supportive experiences and great connections are made," she says, "but there can be some reason for taking caution around those things and really being careful with one's safety."

INTEGRATION THERAPY AND COACHING

Integration therapy and coaching are two of the newest integration techniques that are popping up all over the US.

Although different, the basic idea of integration therapy and coaching are the same: talking to a professional to help you unpack your psychedelic experience. However, the difference is important. Elizabeth Nielson explains that integration therapy, or someone who is advertised as an "integration therapist," is more likely a licensed, clinical professional, either a psychologist or social worker, who has done some kind of professional training on psychedelics and integration, like the course she hosts for professionals.[105] Therefore, these licensed professionals are bound to certain legal standards, like confidentiality and privacy. Coaches, on the other hand, are often unlicensed, and although they may be "wonderfully competent," they are not legally held to the same standards. Nielson gave me an example of when privacy matters: If a therapist's records were to be subpoenaed in divorce court, she would be prepared to fight that to protect her client's privacy. However, a coach might have fewer resources or legal protections to do so. So it's important to ask potential therapists if they're licensed.

Of course there are other differences between coaches and therapists as well. Integration therapy might very well look like normal therapy, a nondirective talking approach to help clients find meaning from psychedelics and other experiences, like childhood memories or dreams. Coaching, on the other hand, might be more directive, and coaches might feel comfortable giving clients more concrete advice on how to enact lessons in the here and now. If you're trying to choose between the two, it will really depend on what kind of support you're looking for and the level of privacy you require. The last crucial difference

---

105   Elizabeth Nielson and Ingmar Gorman, Psychedelic Psychotherapy: Psychedelics for Clinicians 101 & 102.

to mention is that a therapist's time is likely to be reimbursed, at least partially, by your health insurance, while a coach's payment will more likely have to come completely out of pocket.

Yet, do you really need a professional to help you integrate? Nielson points out that no, integration therapy is not necessary for everyone who does a psychedelic. "We don't have any intention of pathologizing psychedelic use by offering integration in the therapy setting," she says. However, she does note that most people who reach out to her for integration therapy often already have a history of depression, anxiety, PTSD, or similar condition, and so for them, an integration therapist gives them the extra support they may need going into and coming out of a psychedelic experience. If you are someone who wants to use psychedelics for healing and dealing with mental health conditions similar to the ones mentioned, enlisting a professional's guidance is a great idea, though it's not a guarantee that psychedelics will be as effective as in clinical trials. However, having an expert's assistance can still be really beneficial for your journey and continued growth and wellness.

If you're considering a psychedelic experience and also an integration professional, Nielson says, ideally, you should schedule your first appointment before your trip. That way, the therapist or coach can help you decide if plant medicine is the best option for you, give you alternative ideas, like float tanks or holotropic breathwork, and also help you prepare mentally and spiritually as well as for any possibly acute and post-trip effects and feelings. Then, after your psychedelic experience (or breathwork session), you'll be more fully prepared to start unpacking and learning from your trip with that same person.

Zelfand explains that her method is all about empowering the person rather than getting too bogged down in what happened during the trip; it's more about what it meant to the individual. "Where does this fit into your sense of yourself as a cohesive human? Where do you want it to fit?" are more the types of questions she has her patients ponder. Nielson's description of her sessions as a private-practice integration psychologist is very similar. "How do they see [their trip] in terms of their longer term trajectory? What's really important about it?" She brings it back to "inner healing wisdom" and explains she encourages people to develop and trust their own intuition about the best way to move forward.

It's important to note: Integration therapists or coaches do not administer psychedelics, do not conduct guided dose sessions, and don't recommend places to buy substances, but they can help you prepare for a safe journey and, obviously, integrate it after the fact. You can find psychedelic integration therapists on the Psychedelic Support Network's website[106] or by using the MAPS database.[107] If there aren't any in your area, therapists who are licensed in your state may also provide sessions online via video conference. Coaches in any location also offer video chat sessions to clients around the country.

---

106   Psychedelic Support. https://psychedelic.support/network/
107   MAPS. https://integration.maps.org.

MINDFULNESS AND MEDITATION

Meditation and other mindfulness techniques are also popular ways to integrate. In fact, a recent clinical trial out of Johns Hopkins showed that people who were taught how to meditate during their course of psychedelic-assisted therapy had the most beneficial experiences compared to groups who only received standard support.[108] If you already have a practice of meditation in your life, great, you're ahead of the curve. But, if you don't, try starting one before your psychedelic experience.

There are lots of different meditation techniques that you can find online, and you can even find guided meditations on YouTube. But for a simple start, the *Psychedelic Times* recommends sitting somewhere comfortable for just five minutes to begin, and focus on your breath. When thoughts come, acknowledge them and try to let them go. The same applies to any physical aches or pains; acknowledge, then let go, like releasing a balloon and watching it disappear into the horizon.[109] Once you get comfortable doing this for five minutes, try it for ten, and even set a timer if it helps. The important thing is to sit quietly with yourself and notice your breath, and then take it from there.

This kind of practice can help you come to new insights regarding your psychedelic experience or ways to apply lessons you've already received. Because a strong mushroom trip can open you up to new ways of thinking about yourself, a meditation practice can help keep you mindful of your behavior and intentions on a regular basis. If you're actively engaging in mindfulness, it'll be

---

108   Griffiths, et al., "Psilocybin-Occasioned Mystical-Type Experience."
109   Psychedelic Times Staff, "Integrating a Psychedelic Experience."

easier to catch yourself acting out of balance with the realizations you had on your journey.

YOGA, EMBODIMENT, AND OTHER BODYWORK TECHNIQUES

Embodiment and other bodywork can take a lot of forms when it comes to psychedelic integration. One of the most popular ways people can work with their bodies after their trip is through yoga, but activities like dance, Tai Chi, and Qigong can also be helpful, as can acupuncture, massage, and even Reiki. The idea here is getting in touch with your body, especially if your trip was particularly physical or difficult to put into words. During a psychedelic experience, there can be a strong sense of feeling your body in a novel way, says Nielson, and so bodywork techniques can help people practice something that brings them back in touch with themselves by focusing on sensations and breath. "These kinds of practices can be very helpful for remembering the differences in the experience of one's physicality," Nielson explains.

Of course, this will also be very individual to the person. Zelfand exemplifies this when she tells me of a woman she knows who used physical therapy as part of her integration. During her psychedelic experience, this woman relived a sexual assault she was the victim of. When she was raped, she was forcibly held down, and she experienced a similar sensation when she was tripping. After her journey, she realized that since her assault, she had been disconnected from her pelvis. Even though she had sexual relationships with people, Zelfand explains, she still didn't feel like she was completely present in her pelvic area. And so, part of this woman's integration was going to see a physical therapist to strengthen her pelvic floor. What's more, during her psychedelic experience, she realized that since being held down during her trauma, she had been holding both her physical body and her emotions down. To reclaim her agency, she signed up for a dance class, rekindling a love she had for dance as a child. Now she goes to dance class every week "and she's got amazing pelvic-floor tone," says Zelfand. This particular woman didn't need to go to talk therapy to figure this stuff out, even though she had a history of a trauma. Zelfand explains, she "got it," she knew she wanted to "nourish herself in those ways now," and physical therapy and dance were how she integrated a distressing but useful psychedelic experience for personal growth.

INSPIRING AWE

Many people recommend going out into nature as a way to integrate, and it is a popular and useful tool. That's because going out into the wilderness can inspire awe, like the kind that you experience during a psychedelic trip. Mother Nature is incredible in its complexity and beauty, and spending time at a local park or hiking in the woods can be extremely useful in reconnecting to that experience of incomprehensible beauty and things greater than yourself. This can be beneficial the days immediately following your psychedelic journey, as can continuing to spend more time somewhere that you can quietly reflect, relax, and take in greatness. While obviously nature is a wonderful place to inspire awe and unwind, letting emotions or possible insights come to you, it's not the only place that elicits that "small self" feeling. Listening to music from your trip can also help, as can going to other places that provoke reverence, like a museum, a live concert, play or other type of performance, or whatever inspires you personally. Maybe that's street art, maybe that's traveling to a foreign country, or maybe it's taking time to look up at the stars at night. It could be reading a great book or skydiving; going to a ballet, planetarium, or musical. Again, this all comes back to your intuition. There's no right or wrong way to inspire awe, and it'll be individual to what stirs you. The important thing is to go somewhere that moves you to reflect on things grander than yourself and that inspires the same feeling of amazement that you're an important part of such a complex and beautiful world.

CONTINUE READING AND RESEARCHING

Lastly, many people are comforted during their integration by reading about other people's experiences, both psychedelic, mystical, and beyond. A man in his early 30s, who occasionally uses macrodoses of mushrooms for personal growth, told me that reading about psychedelic science, other "trip lit," and even related topics like philosophy and psychology helped to put his sometimes-confusing and scary psychedelic experiences into perspective. Especially if your trip has you feeling a bit isolated and alone, reading about others' journeys, either in books, articles, or online message boards, can help you to feel like part of something and to deconstruct your experience.

WHAT A POST-PSYCHEDELIC EXPERIENCE CAN LOOK LIKE

Before concluding this chapter, I wanted to go over some common post-trip feelings so you don't worry in the days and weeks following a psychedelic journey. Mainly, it's completely normal to feel a bit stirred up. This depends on the person, the substance, and the experience, but feeling a bit unsettled or raw is totally normal, both Nielson and Zelfand confirm. Being "stirred up" can look a lot of different ways: It could be heightened emotionality, or feeling really raw or very open. Some people describe an afterglow in the day and week after a psilocybin experience, which can be a very positive feeling, but not everyone reacts in the same way. What's more, once the afterglow wears off, people can then begin to feel this stirred up sensation and fear that they're worse off than before. But that's often not the case, and rather, it's all part of the psychedelic process that's still unraveling. Nielson explains that a big part of her job as an integration therapist is to evaluate people to see if they can still care for themselves despite feeling unusually emotional. And if they can, she emphasizes to clients that this feeling will pass. She explains it's important not to pathologize people's feelings further and increase their anxiety.

Plus, both Nielson and Zelfand explain that a heightened emotionality after a psychedelic experience can even be beneficial. "Just because something's stirred up isn't necessarily bad," says Nielson. "People may be experiencing things that they were shut down to...The stirring up is what allows the dust to settle into a new way of being that may be much better for the person than the way things were before. But the stirring up is part of the process. It's not an unwanted negative side effect." Zelfand echoes this sentiment, saying this feeling can even resemble a sort of "hypo-mania" for some that can be just the push they need to start making changes in their lives. "I think it's actually a potent therapeutic tool," Zelfand says. "You're realizing like, wow, I've really got to join a gym and start working out; I've got to reach out to my friends and invest in meaningful social relationships. If you're a little manic for a couple of weeks, that can really help you actually take that step of going and joining the gym, or actually picking up the phone and calling your sister, going to have dinner with your grandmother, whatever it is, you start walking in that routine."

Dealing with those post-psychedelic-experience emotions can be hard, especially if you had some profound realizations during your trip or saw how much work you really need to do for personal growth, healing, and integration. But, "it's the work that gives life meaning," says Richards. "The purpose of life isn't just to be happy, but it's to find meaning, to participate in something that's unfolding that maybe is the evolution of consciousness."

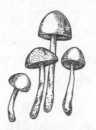

Chapter 12

HOLDING SPACE: HOW TO TRIP SIT

A trip sitter is a sober person you trust to keep you safe while you're under the influence of a psychedelic, and having one along for the journey can make the difference between a meaningful and challenging trip. With a supportive presence, you're much more likely to release your control to the mushrooms and have an insightful, perhaps even transformational experience. Trip sitters are especially handy for your first few psychedelic experiences, or if you're planning on taking a moderate to high dose. Yet, many people prefer to have them for all their psychedelic experiences. But how do you trip sit? Are there any special requirements?

HOW TO PREPARE TO TRIP SIT

Trip sitting is fairly simple. The most important thing to remember is to be a calm, nonjudgmental, and kind presence for the entirety of someone else's psychedelic journey. It's helpful for trip sitters to have psychedelic experience of their own, especially with challenging trips, but this is not completely necessary. Having that firsthand knowledge can help sitters be more empathetic—without becoming anxious—to the weird range of possible sensations that trippers may go through, but preparing yourself by reading guides like this one can also be enough.

Trip sitting is often referred to as "holding space," although the expression isn't exclusive to psychedelics. "Holding space is just being with somebody and allowing them to go through whatever process they need to, without really trying to interfere," says Jessica Grotfeldt, experienced trip sitter and founder of Luz Eterna Psilocybin Retreats. It's really just being present for someone, listening or sitting with them in silence, without offering your opinion or any kind of advice.

So how do you get started? First of all, it's important to have a conversation before the psychedelic experience with the person you're going to be sitting. You'll want to discuss expectations, intentions, boundaries, and to set a loose plan so nothing comes as a surprise. If you've had a psychedelic experience before, but the person you're sitting for has not, talk in depth about how mushrooms can make people feel, both mentally and physically. Some experienced sitters even make people "what to expect" fact sheets, but referring them to Chapter 8 of this book would also suffice! Be sure to also discuss the tripper's intentions: Why do they want to take mushrooms? What do they hope to see, experience, or learn? Discuss any fears or worries they might have and how you plan to deal with any challenging material that might arise. For instance, if the person is afraid they might have a bad trip or be faced with some challenging thoughts or memories, tell them you'll be there to hold their hand and be a shoulder to cry on if they need.

It can also be helpful to discuss a loose plan for the trip day. Talk about the location where the experience will take place. If they're planning on taking mushrooms at their home, ask if anyone else will be there: Are any roommates expected to return home during the trip? Any chance of anyone else showing up that you, as the sitter, may have to deal with? If they don't have any outdoor space at their house, perhaps you want to discuss the possibility of driving to a nearby park or beach toward the end of the experience to connect with nature? It's also important to negotiate difficult issues, like boundaries, ideally days before the experience. While physical touch can really be helpful for those going through a tough time, be sure to discuss it first and set any guidelines. The key is to make everything as transparent as possible to limit surprises on trip day and let voyagers focus on their experience without lingering feelings of uncertainty.

Grotfeldt says it's also crucial to ask if the person you're going to sit with is on any medications or has any chronic medical conditions. Health considerations like diabetes or history of low blood pressure shouldn't prevent you from sitting for someone, but should definitely be discussed and planned for. For example, having medications or some sugary drinks around, like Gatorade, should be planned ahead, in the case of sitting a diabetic. It's also important to know if they have any history of depression or anxiety, and if they're on any medications to treat it. For example, SSRI antidepressants will lessen the effects of psilocybin, even if the tripper skipped that day's dose. While depression and anxiety aren't reasons to cancel sitting a trip, if the person you'll be sitting for explains a history of violent or dissociative behavior, or a more serious personality disorder diagnosis, then you're in more sensitive territory. In these cases, it's best you have a lot of sitting experience or perhaps refer them to a professional guide. Other conditions that are considered dangerous to combine with psychedelics include history of seizures and cardiovascular disease. More information on who should take extra precaution with psychedelics and other possible drug interactions can be found in Chapter 14.

One other way to prepare before the psychedelic experience begins is to have a "backup sitter," recommends Grotfeldt. While it's not necessary to have two sitters for one tripping person, telling someone you trust what you'll be doing can be crucial if an emergency situation arises. While sitters have to be prepared to call emergency services as a last resort if something seriously dangerous goes down, sometimes all you need is a backup sitter to support you and help you think of solutions from another perspective. Another situation where a backup sitter could come in handy is if you're sitting for someone who is physically much larger than you, and they begin to act violently (breaking things, screaming). In this case, you'll want to have a backup sitter on call who is large enough to help the voyager work through these feelings. Basically, having someone to call or text when things get questionable can help you to make the safest choices for those you're sitting.

Lastly, it's important to set aside enough time to trip sit. Medium to high doses of psilocybin generally last at least six hours, with the experience coming on and off in waves toward the end. Therefore, be sure to be available for closer to eight to nine hours to fully support the person you're sitting for. You'll be able to tell when their experience is winding down, but they'll likely still be in a vulnerable and sensitive place. So stick around, help them cook or order some takeout if they're getting their appetite back, and continue to hold space for them. Let them talk it out if they want, or help them settle into a nice nature documentary or other entertainment of their choice. If they're a really close friend, consider spending the night with them or at the very least make yourself available to talk on the phone or via text that night and the next day.

TRIP DAY: TRIP-SITTING ESSENTIALS

On trip day your main job is to stay calm, supportive, and present. Trippers are extra sensitive to the environment, including your mood, so remaining centered and smiling at them when you make eye contact helps. Don't act bored, annoyed, or upset (even if you are) because it can grossly affect their experience for the worse. Many experienced sitters recommend bringing a book so you have something peaceful to do and you're not repeatedly checking your phone. In fact, some sitters recommend wearing a watch so you don't need to take out your phone to check the time. While you are there for the person going on a psychedelic journey, don't completely ignore your own needs. Eat when you're hungry and go to the bathroom when you have to because, again, the tripper will be able to sense when you're uncomfortable and that could cause them to feel uncomfortable.

It's also important to remember that you are not there to guide their trip in any particular direction, but rather to be a nondirective source of support. "Number one, the mushrooms are the teachers," says experienced sitter and founder of The Buena Vida Psilocybin Retreats Amanda Schendel. "We are not there to counsel or guide someone in a specific direction or to ask them pointed questions. We're just there to keep everyone physically and emotionally safe and to be a support if someone needs it. So I train people to speak as little as possible and to never insert themselves into someone's experience." If someone wants to talk, listen, smile, nod, put your arm around them, offer them a tissue if they're tearing up, but don't give advice or anything too opinionated.

It's also crucial never to be condescending or patronizing in any way. Don't talk to trippers like they're children or like they're stupid because that can really send people into a negative place. If they're your close friends, talk to them as you normally would, perhaps more sparingly. It's also common for trippers to want to be left alone, and that's totally fine. It absolutely doesn't mean they don't need you anymore and you can leave, because having someone around that's sober, who they can trust, will still be a pillar of support. Instead, discuss this the day before. Tell them it's common to want some alone time, but if that happens, suggest they go into another room and leave the door ajar so you can periodically check in on them without disturbing them.

However, sometimes when trippers are alone, they can go through some of their most difficult inner material. When you poke your head in to check on them, you'll be able to tell if they need some support by their breathing. If their chest is going up and down rapidly, they're probably struggling, and it's a good time to sit next to them and just hold their hand. You might not even have to say anything, but often a supportive, gentle touch can go a long way. People may not communicate their needs because they're too far gone, so you can ask, or just offer them things like a thick blanket, a glass of water, some tissues, or just a hand to hold.

People may also need help with things like going to the bathroom or getting up to walk around because their bodies feel so differently. Everyday things can be a struggle, like changing the music or putting on a movie or video games, so if they express interest in one of these activities, offer to set it up for them. Even adjusting the volume of music or the brightness of lights can be difficult when on mushrooms, so that's your job as trip sitter.

HOW TO HELP SOMEONE THROUGH A CHALLENGING TRIP

Likely, the most difficult thing you'll encounter as a sitter is helping someone through an emotionally challenging experience. As we've been discussing in this book, mushrooms can bring up distressing emotions, past traumas, unresolved guilt, or grief among a host of other tough and even otherworldly experiences. But resisting these inner struggles only makes a challenging trip more difficult. That's why *The Manual of Psychedelic Support* recommends that sitters talk trippers through these challenging experiences rather than talking them down or out of them. In fact, the Multidisciplinary Association for Psychedelic Studies (MAPS) teaches sitters to encourage trippers to "explore all emotions, even difficult ones." Once trippers relax and let all of their emotions flow, they'll stop resisting the experience and likely find incredible insights, deep inner peace, or even transcendence on the other side.[110]

The best thing a sitter can do for a tripper going through a difficult experience is to just be there for them. Sit down next to them and only talk if they want to. Again, physical touch might help, so hold their hand or touch their shoulder if you've already discussed beforehand this is something they're comfortable with. Offer them a blanket to snuggle under, some tissues, or a glass of water. Make eye contact, smile, and act empathetic and understanding, not worried or concerned (even if you actually are). Grotfeldt tells me the best thing you can do for someone having a challenging trip or even a panic attack is to help them connect with their breath. Take deep breaths with them and if they're able, try doing some simple breathwork. Grotfeldt recommends pranayama breathing, which is inhaling for three seconds, holding for six, and exhaling for nine. Count for them gently and hold their hand if they want. Grotfeldt also tells me it can help to have trippers take their shoes off and touch their feet to the ground while breathing deeply. If they're really struggling with something and don't want to sit with it, suggest taking a little walk, even if it's around the room. "People just need to

---

110   MAPS, "How to Work with Difficult Experiences."

move their energy in a way that helps distract them," Grotfeldt says. "If they're unable to walk, breathing with their feet on the ground and reminding them that you're there and that you're taking care of their physical body helps."

Sometimes a challenging experience looks more like a person being very confused. People can forget who and where they are or think they're dying or going crazy. Trippers can also get paranoid and might project this onto their sitter, thinking you're talking about them, conspiring against them, or that you even tried to poison them. The key is to remain calm and kind in all situations. If people are very confused, using their first name when you talk to them can really help. If they think they're dying or going crazy, remind them that they took magic mushrooms and that the effects will begin to wear off soon, and of course, that you're there for them no matter what.

Sometimes people on mushrooms get stuck in negative thought loops that are hard to get themselves out of or resolve. So if you notice this as a sitter, you can try to introduce some distractions like beautiful, colorful, or sparkly things to look at together. You could try to watch a nature documentary together, go for a little walk, or get up and move the body by shaking or dancing. The classic recommendations are to change the scenery, music, or lighting; these alterations can help change a tripper's mood quickly. Do an activity together if they want, like making art or banging on a percussive instrument. The best thing you can do is to remain calm, centered, chill, and friendly. Don't get stressed or anxious or try to fix everything. Sometimes people just need to cry it out for a while, and it's a very healing and cathartic experience. Don't make a big deal of anything, even if they spill something on you, throw up, or wet their pants. Just remind them it's all part of the experience and help them clean up while remaining positive.

Trip-Sitting Basics

Do:

- Be supportive yet nondirective.

- Be soft-spoken and gentle.

- Smile and make eye contact.

- Be understanding and kind.

- Be willing to talk but more willing to listen.

- Be willing to change and turn music on or off (and always respect their choices).

- Help with movies, video games, lights, and handle other electronics and technical tasks.

- Get snacks and drinks. Order pizza or help make food toward the end.

- Offer tissues, blankets, and distractions if you feel they're needed.

- Be willing to call emergency services as a last resort.

Don't:

- Be condescending, aggressive, annoyed, or stressed.

- Bring up negative, tough memories or emotional topics.

- Dismiss anything they say as worthless, stupid, immature, or "just the drugs talking."

- Ask them if they're feeling it, how they feel, or probe them about anything too often.

- Make a big deal if they have an accident, spill or break something, cry, talk too loudly, have a hard time, throw up, etc.

- Have other drugs on you in public.

- Ignore them or leave before the trip concludes.

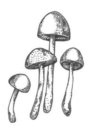

Chapter 13

MICRODOSING MUSHROOMS

Microdosing is all the rage, and possibly how magic mushrooms and LSD will go fully mainstream. Since James Fadiman publicly coined the term in 2011,[III] there have been thousands of articles on the topic as well as podcasts, YouTube videos, popular subreddits, and first-person accounts on social media. Yet, what's still lacking—at the time of writing this book—are any controlled, double-blind scientific studies, the gold standard in testing the safety and efficacy of novel medications. While Fadiman writes indigenous cultures have been using microdoses of mind-expanding plant medicines for centuries, probably millennia, Western science is still far behind. However, with thousands of people experimenting with microdosing psychedelics around the globe at this very moment for a host of reasons, it's important to

---

III   Fadiman, *The Psychedelic Explorer's Guide.*

get familiar with what is known and the little research that has been done, in order to decide if microdosing is right for you.

WHAT IS A MICRODOSE?

A microdose is one-tenth to one-twentieth of a recreational dose of psychedelics. In terms of psilocybin mushrooms, that's anywhere from 0.1 to 0.5 grams of dried material. The key to microdosing is taking so little that you barely notice it. Often referred to as a "sub-perceptual" dose, microdosers feel a little different on microdose days, usually characterized by an elated mood or feeling energized, according to Fadiman and his research partner, Sophia Krob.[112] However, the researchers add that you shouldn't feel any of the classic psychedelic sensory changes. In fact, if you do start to see things breathe or begin tripping slightly, this is considered an overdose in the microdose world and is regarded as the main possible negative side effect.

WHY DO PEOPLE MICRODOSE?

"I wanted to get off SSRIs," a 51-year-old singer-songwriter told me. "I quit drinking seven years ago, but I still wanted a social lubricant of some kind," a 33-year-old CEO said. "After my teenage son died, my rage was out of control. I was afraid I was going to kill someone," a 62-year-old man revealed to me over the phone. "I thought about killing myself every day," a 28-year-old grad student told me on the Signal app. "My depression and

---

112   Fadiman and Krob, "Microdosing Psychedelics."

IBS were so bad it was hard to get out of bed in the morning," a 31-year-old man, whose mom connected us, confided.

Microdosers are everywhere, and they're more than the techy Silicon Valley trope that's been recently popularized.[113] What I've found is they're often people with depression, anxiety, or PTSD that's threatening to take over their lives. But in microdosing, they've found a solution. That's not to say this will work for everyone, and if you're seriously depressed, don't go off your medication and start microdosing without consulting your doctor. But it does seem to help a wide range of people without producing a full-blown trip, and so there's less need to control and plan for set, setting, and all the other considerations discussed in this book. Fadiman and Krob have also reported that folks with treatment-resistant depression are the majority of people who reach out to them. It's not surprising, considering depression is the number-one cause of disability worldwide.[114] People are desperate for answers, and they're willing to break the law and microdose if it proves fruitful.

However, it's not just anecdotal reports on the benefits of microdosing for depression, scientific studies are starting to back up these claims too. A 2019 study by Polito, et al. found reduced levels of reported long-term depression and stress, as well as feeling more connected, contemplative, creative, focused, and productive in the short term on actual microdose days.[115] Similarly, in a 2018 paper by Anderson, et al., researchers found microdosers had lower levels of "dysfunctional attitudes"

113   Solon, "Under Pressure, Silicon Valley."

114   According to the World Health Organization (WHO). https://www.who.int/news-room/fact-sheets/detail/depression

115   Polito, et al., "A Systematic Study of Microdosing."

than non-microdosers, which, according to the authors, is an indicator of lower depression and vulnerability to stressors. They also tested microdosers and found them to experience less negative emotionality, which includes depression and anxiety, yet they cautioned that more research needs to be done before drawing any conclusions on microdosing's effects on depression.[116] However, this is in line with many anecdotal reports. Or, in the words of Fadiman and Krob, "Simply put, people felt more up and less down."

Yet all sorts of people, not limited to those who struggle with mental health, are experimenting with microdosing for many different reasons. For instance, increased creativity and productivity are highly reported reasons in the media, and now there's some preliminary research to support this claim. Of the very few studies there are on microdosing psychedelics, a recent paper found that both convergent and divergent thinking—both indicators of creativity—improved after microdosing psilocybin-containing truffles (which are legal in the Netherlands, where the study was performed).[117]

As far as productivity goes, people are claiming microdosing has become a replacement for other concentration and work-enhancement drugs like caffeine, Adderall, or Ritalin.[118] While it's highly contested among microdosers, there is some initial research to support this claim as well. For instance, in the 2019 Polito, et al. paper mentioned above, researchers found microdosers had "significant reductions in mind wandering," which has implications for concentration and has also been

---

116   Anderson, et al., "Microdosing Psychedelics: Personality, Mental Health."
117   Prochazkova, et al., "Exploring the Effect of Microdosing Psychedelics."
118   Smith, "Meet the People Who."

linked to "greater levels of happiness" according to the authors. Yet at the same time, some microdosers I spoke to reported that productivity can really depend on the activity. For instance, Stephanie (name changed for privacy) told me she could get lost in creative endeavors, like writing poetry or working on her often-neglected Etsy store, but working in front of a computer all day was tough. She explained that once she learned how she reacted to microdosing, she would adjust her schedule to make sure she didn't have any mundane tasks to complete on a microdose day because she found it more challenging than on off days.

People also report microdose effects that are more in line with how we think of the mind-expanding qualities of psychedelics. For example, people observe being more empathetic—a common quality of higher mushroom doses—as well as more able to live in the present moment and being more in tune with one's real needs.[119] And research is beginning to support these claims as well. For instance, in the 2018 Anderson, et al. study, researchers tested microdosers and found them to score higher on "open-mindedness," which they hypothesized considering recent findings on increased openness with higher-dose sessions.[120] They also found microdosers to score higher on tests of "wisdom," which they defined as being able to "reflect learning from one's mistakes, consider multiple perspectives when facing a situation, being in tune with one's emotions and those of others, and feeling a sense of connection and unity." For those of us who have gained incredible insight and perspective from higher-dose mushroom experiences, it's not surprising

---

119   Passie, *The Science of Microdosing Psychedelics.*

120   MacLean, et al., "Mystical Experiences Occasioned by the Hallucinogen."

that microdoses may imbue some of those qualities to users as well.

What's more, people are even reporting relief from cluster headaches and migraines, which is another area of interest psychedelic scientists are looking into with both high and micro doses.[121] Some are using microdosing to help them cut back on other substances, like cigarettes, cannabis, kratom, coffee, and alcohol, as well as prescription medications like Adderall, Klonopin, and Zoloft. People even use microdosing as a social lubricant and more natural replacement for other party drugs like alcohol and cocaine. That's because microdosing can be energizing and great for late-night dancing, as well as anxiety reducing, making it fun at a party or networking event. Dan, a young CEO who uses microdoses socially told me he even likes to take 0.25 grams before a rich meal with friends to enhance the flavors, textures, and conversations.

While it seems like microdosing may be a serious option to consider, in *The Science of Microdosing Psychedelics*, Torsten Passie warns that it seems like microdosing is a "kind of panacea to cope with all the problems a modern American confronts at her workplace or in their personal life. It seems highly probable that most of these claims, especially those mentioned one or a very few times, are not based on factual changes, but more on a wishful thinking, placebo responses, or lively imagination."

So could microdosing's positively glowing potential all come down to the placebo effect? Considering it's very likely microdoses of psilocybin interact with the brain's serotonin system in a similar fashion to high doses—by increasing neuroplasticity and

---

121   Sewell, et al., "Response of Cluster Headache to Psilocybin and LSD."

quieting the Default Mode Network[122] (see Chapter 4 for more detail)—it seems unlikely, in my opinion, that microdosing is nothing more than a placebo. However, there are, at the time of writing this book, no studies on the neurophysiological effects of microdoses, and as Passie points out in his book, "We also don't know *how much* of a psychedelic substance is needed to increase neuroplasticity."[123] And, hypothetically, if microdoses aren't affecting the brain in a similar way to full doses, and all of these claimed microdose effects are just placebo, would that be so bad? Maybe not, especially considering the 2008 finding that most of the effects from legal antidepressants are actually "based on placebo effects" as well.[124] Furthermore, James Giordano explains that some people are more suggestible, and "taking something at a low dose actually allows them to engender their own *physiological* responses to change their perception of certain things." He emphasizes that the placebo response isn't phony, it just means that for certain people, suggestion is enough for them to actually "change some of their [brain] network activity," imbuing the results they hope to achieve in microdosing themselves—unconsciously.

HOW TO MICRODOSE

The crux to microdosing is that it doesn't interfere with your daily routine. In fact, it's recommended by the Fadiman protocol (that we explain below) to go about your day as usual, including work, meals, sleep, and even medications. Of course, if you

---

122   Carhart-Harris and Friston, "REBUS and the Anarchic Brain."

123   Passie, *The Science of Microdosing Psychedelics.*

124   Kirsch, et al., "Initial Severity and Antidepressant Benefits."

accidentally overdose and start feeling substantial psychedelic effects, driving to work might be dangerous and focusing on a computer screen might seem impossible, but that's why you have to be sure to weigh out your dose. It might also be a good move to experiment with microdosing for the first time on a weekend or a day where you have fewer responsibilities to get a good sense of how it makes you feel.

In order to microdose, the first thing you have to do is weigh out your dried mushrooms. Most people use a kitchen or jewelry scale to do so. You can buy one for around 10 to 15 dollars online, just make sure it can read measurements as little as 0.1 grams (100 milligrams) or less. For your first microdose, start small. Weigh out 0.1 grams and take it in the morning. Remember, just because you're taking less than a full dose doesn't mean it will last a shorter amount of time, so unless you want it to keep you up in the evening, take it early in the day to avoid a restless night. Finding your personal perfect dose will take some trial and error, so on the first microdose day, start very small and see how it makes you feel. After finding out how your body reacts to the microdose, then you can experiment with different doses. Try going up to 0.2 grams and evaluate your physical and mental sensations. Many people seem to benefit from a dose around 0.25 to 0.3 grams while others prefer even smaller, around 0.12. It'll be different for every individual. Plus, mushrooms vary in strength, which can make microdosing a little tricky. For example, if you've been very comfortable microdosing 0.3 grams, but you run out and buy, grow, or pick a new batch, 0.3 might feel a little different. So start small again or test them on a day when you have less to do just in case you overdose slightly.

THE FADIMAN PROTOCOL

James Fadiman developed a suggested microdosing protocol[125] that Ayelet Waldman used in her funny and informative book on microdosing LSD, *A Really Good Day*.[126] It's basically a schedule of when to take your microdose in order to avoid any kind of tolerance buildup.

Day One: Microdose

Day Two: Off day (where many people report still feeling really good)

Day Three: Off day (to get it totally out of your system)

Day Four: Microdose again

Fadiman suggests people microdose in this way for no more than a month or two while keeping track of their moods, productivity, and other feelings and sensations in a daily journal. While many microdosers who I interviewed for this book had heard of the protocol, most of them didn't follow it very strictly. Some tried it for a few weeks or months, then either stopped completely or adjusted to microdose more infrequently, like a few times a month. Others, including two men I interviewed who found great relief from previous mental distress with microdosing psilocybin, microdosed every day for over six months without any noticeable negative side effects or tolerance buildup. Both of these men told me that non-microdose days were too difficult because their symptoms came back in full force. At the moment, there is no research on the long-term use of microdoses, but

---

125   Fadiman's microdosing website: microdosingpsychedelics.com.
126   Waldman, *A Really Good Day*.

both of my interviewees were more concerned about what they might do when they weren't microdosing than what might happen if they continued on a daily basis.

POSSIBLE NEGATIVE SIDE EFFECTS, OR DRUG INTERACTIONS

Like with any medicine, microdosing psilocybin isn't for everyone, and there are some possible adverse reactions. The most common negative side effect—aside from accidentally taking too much—is trouble sleeping on microdose days. There are also reports of some mild gastrointestinal upset, like nausea or appetite loss, from microdosing. But a 31-year-old I spoke with told me that microdosing psilocybin daily actually increases his appetite and helps to regulate his constant gastro upset caused by his irritable bowel syndrome (IBS).

While many have found relief from social and general anxiety by microdosing, others have found the opposite, that they experience mild anxiety instead.[127] Similarly, while many have found microdosing helps them with impulse control and irritability,[128] others have found that it can increase their irritability, especially if they've taken a little too much or during off days. What's more, some people benefit from microdosing's apparent empathy-enhancing qualities, but others have found they can become too emotionally sensitive on microdose days. Likewise, the 2019 Polito, et al. study mentioned above also

---

127   Reddit forum, "Negative Experiences."
128   Waldman, *A Really Good Day.*

had a finding that wasn't glowingly positive: microdosers scored higher on tests of neuroticism. The researchers point out that an increase in neuroticism may actually "reflect an overall increase in the intensity of emotions (both positive and negative) experienced during periods of microdosing. Reports of intense emotions were common in participants' comments... It may be that as participants become less distracted (i.e., experience reduced mind wandering) and more absorbed in their immediate experience, they are more able to identify and process negative emotions." As someone who's reported on cannabis's medical benefits for years before investigating mushrooms, I found this very similar to different people's reactions to weed. For some, it's a godsend for anxiety; for others, it's a panic attack in a plant. Neither cannabis nor psilocybin are a "one size fits all" medication, but in reality, not many prescription drugs (especially those used for depression) are either.

But is there anyone who definitely shouldn't microdose? After reviewing over 1,000 self-reports on microdosing, Fadiman and Krob have identified some conditions that don't mix well with the practice. For one, they've found those with red-green color blindness experience "lasting visual distortions," and so they don't recommend those people dabble. Similar to the precautions against high-dose psychedelics, they also caution those who live with psychosis to avoid microdosing so they don't aggravate their condition. Additionally, they also advise against pregnant people microdosing, only because there's no research on the subject yet.[129]

As far as possible drug interactions, there are no official studies. However, while collecting user reports, Fadiman and Krob

129   Microdosing Psychedelics, "FAQ on Microdosing."

compiled a list of medications people have mixed without adverse reactions, which you can find on their site.[130] One drug they have had a negative report of is lithium. Fadiman and Krob received an account from a woman who said mixing microdosing and lithium made her very dizzy "to the point where she couldn't stand."[131] I would also exercise caution when mixing SSRI antidepressants and microdoses of psilocybin because they both affect the serotonin system in the brain. While an adverse reaction combining SSRIs with a microdose isn't likely according to Fadiman's site, as we'll discuss in Chapter 14, these kinds of antidepressants can lessen the effects of full-dose psychedelics and will likely do the same with microdoses.

I would also be cautious about mixing microdoses of psilocybin with cannabis. While many regular cannabis consumers don't feel any different when combining the two, people with a low cannabis tolerance or those who get anxious after using high-THC cannabis might have increased anxiety when mixing it with a microdose of psilocybin. We'll also discuss this in more depth in Chapter 14, but cannabis and psilocybin can enhance each other's effects, which can be a complement for some but overwhelming and anxiety inducing for others. It's not that the combo should absolutely be avoided, but extra caution should be taken.

130 Microdosing Psychedelics, "Drugs and Supplements."
131 Fadiman and Krob, "Microdosing Psychedelics."

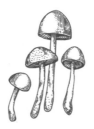

Chapter 14

THE POTENTIAL RISKS OF PSILOCYBIN

There's a lot of talk about how psychedelics aren't for everyone, that maybe some people should avoid "mind revealing" substances like psilocybin due to preexisting mental or physical health conditions. It's a controversial topic in the psychedelic community, with anecdotes proving both sides of the story. At first I thought to call this chapter "Who should avoid psychedelics?" but changed the wording because it's not exactly true. When I asked experts about the conditions we're going to look at in this chapter, most told me there could be instances of these people using psilocybin, just under much more controlled settings than your average "naturalistic" mushroom trip. So while this chapter is meant to give you information to make an informed decision, there are no hard and fast rules on who should and shouldn't take magic mushrooms.

Yet even Terence McKenna, one of the biggest proponents of taking psychedelics, believed they weren't for everyone. In an interview with *OMNI* magazine in 1993, he responded to the question, "What people specifically should not take them?" like this: "People who are mentally unstable, under enormous pressure, or operating equipment that the lives of hundreds of people depend on. Or the fragile ones among us—those to whom you wouldn't give a weekend airline ticket to Paris, those who wouldn't expect to guide you out of the Yukon. Some people have been so damaged by life that boundary dissolution is not helpful to them. These people are trying to maintain boundaries, their functionality. They should be honored and supported, and not encouraged to take drugs. If because of genetic or cultural or psychological factors it's not for you, then it's not for you."[132]

WHO'S DISQUALIFIED FROM PARTICIPATING IN CLINICAL TRIALS AND WHY?

For whom do psychedelics pose the biggest risk? To answer this question, I looked at what types of conditions disqualify people from participating in clinical trials with psilocybin. At the moment, the main conditions include hypertension and other underlying heart conditions; history of psychosis or a psychotic spectrum disorder like schizophrenia; bipolar disorder; other persistent severe mental illness; as well as a first-degree relative

---

132   *OMNI,* "Terence McKenna Interview."

with any of these psychiatric conditions. Also, for the time being, pregnant people are also excluded.

However, three active psychedelic researchers I spoke with all expressed a desire to work with most of these populations in the future. Therefore, it's not that people with these conditions absolutely cannot take psychedelics. But the risks are greater, as we're about to explain in the next sections, and so there will likely be more of a need for trained guides, thorough preparation, and close post-session monitoring. Ros Watts explains simply that their trials are essentially rushed at the moment, and there's not enough time to give these populations the extra support they might require. Peter Hendricks has a different take, "If something were to go wrong at these early stages, psilocybin would likely be blamed as the cause for that negative outcome." Essentially, Hendricks believes researchers are taking an abundance of caution in order to ensure psychedelic research can continue without hiccups like they encountered in the 1960s. He explains, in his other research on smoking cessation, if his team were doing a large clinical trial with a new nicotine patch, they would sadly anticipate a few fatalities just due to the population. Some might be older, smoking for decades, and their deaths are a potential reality that wouldn't immediately be blamed on the nicotine patch they were testing. But with the heightened political lens surrounding psilocybin trials, if anything went wrong, he believes it could potentially threaten the whole future of psychedelic research.

All that being said, if you do have one of the following conditions, please seriously weigh the potential risks and benefits of using psilocybin, and don't go into a psychedelic experience without adequate preparation and support for both the drug experience and the weeks following.

HYPERTENSION AND OTHER UNDERLYING HEART CONDITIONS

The main physical condition researchers screen for in clinical trials with psychedelics is hypertension. Erica Zelfand explains that because psilocybin affects serotonin pathways, it can transiently run the risk of elevating blood pressure and altering body temperature. Hendricks elaborates, explaining that psilocybin can modestly increase blood pressure, "by maybe 20 points. If you have an underlying heart condition, like serious arrhythmia or you are hypertensive, it can create a condition in which the likelihood of a heart event is raised." He says that he "wouldn't be surprised" that a high dose of psilocybin could cause a heart attack in someone with a heart condition, "But then so could exercise, so could a number of things, right?" He adds that, for these people, taking psilocybin would "at least require physician oversight and monitoring."

There also seems to be extra risk for those who have had a past open-heart surgery. One of the only recorded deaths associated with psilocybin ingestion was of a heart transplant recipient.[133] This person received a heart transplant 10 years before her psilocybin experience, but it was apparently still too much for

---

133   Lim, et al., "A Fatal Case of 'Magic Mushroom.'"

her body to handle, and she went into cardiac arrest two to three hours after consuming mushrooms.[134]

PSYCHOTIC SPECTRUM DISORDERS

The main mental health condition the psychedelic community warns people about is schizophrenia or a family history of a psychotic spectrum disorder. It's generally believed that taking a psychedelic when you are genetically predisposed to experience psychosis can speed along the time of your first psychotic break, and Hendricks confirms this for me in so many words. For this same reason he says it's especially dangerous for young people with a predisposition to psychosis to take psilocybin.

When I ask Watts about this, she points me to a study from the mid-twentieth century, where a participant had a "problematic psychotic response" to LSD. When it was investigated further, it was found that this person was the twin brother of someone with schizophrenia, and so now these types of first-degree relatives are excluded to prevent this from reoccurring. Obviously more research is needed moving forward. "It's not conclusive," says Hendricks. "I even think there could be a future in which we examine psilocybin as a treatment for schizophrenia because it involves obviously affective disturbance and depression, and I think there might be a case for that."

---

134   Erowid.org, "Psilocybin Mushrooms: Fatalities/Deaths."

BIPOLAR DISORDER

Bipolar disorder is another condition that can disqualify people from currently participating in clinical trials, but it's also another controversial and multilayered topic. There's a sort of understanding in the psychedelic community that someone with bipolar disorder or a family history of bipolar disorder could be thrust into a manic episode following a psychedelic experience. Zelfand explains that it would be unethical to do a study testing this theory, but pointed out the main concern is for those who have bipolar 1 disorder, which is characterized by manic highs and depressive lows. Those with bipolar 2, on the other hand, who don't experience manic episodes, would be at a lower risk, she thinks. Watts also confirms this when I asked her why people with the disorder were disqualified, but reiterates she doesn't think psychedelics are completely off-limits to these folk. However, they might need extra support that her team cannot provide at the moment.

Hendricks answers slightly differently. He explains his team excludes folks with bipolar as an extra precaution ensuring those with a genetic disposition to psychosis don't get into the study. "Sometimes people with psychosis get misdiagnosed as having bipolar disorder," he explains, "because mania and psychosis can look so similar."

The bottom line for those with bipolar or a family history of the condition is precaution. Especially if it's bipolar 1, and you've had a history of dangerous manic episodes, psilocybin poses an extra risk, and you may need a knowledgeable and open-minded psychiatrist in place to support you in the weeks following your trip. What's more, if you're already medicated for bipolar disorder, there are potential risks of mixing your medication with psilocybin (which I'll explain below), and of course, it's inadvisable to go off your medication without a doctor's supervision. This all being said, hopefully, in the future, there will be legal psychedelic therapy options that can provide the extra support that those who live with this disorder may need.

OTHER MENTAL HEALTH CONCERNS

When I ask researchers if there is anyone else disqualified from their trials for the time being, Hendricks explains they're excluding people with "severe persistent mental illness." He admits it's out of an abundance of caution, but the worry is that psilocybin could exacerbate that person's underlying psychiatric condition.

Watts tells me there's another group that's currently excluded from her study: those who struggle to form trusting bonds with the therapists in a short amount of time. She explains that's often people with borderline personality disorder and other personality disorders, who struggle to trust others and regulate their emotions. "And of course they can [form trusting bonds], but it often takes a bit longer. And in our study, it's so rushed that we're asking people to come in and trust us very quickly and go into this potentially very difficult stuff with someone they don't know. Somebody with a personality disorder might just struggle to do that," Watts says.

One last exclusion criteria for some of the current clinical trials includes a "history of serious suicide attempts (requiring hospitalization)."[135] This is, again, an extra precaution to ensure participants don't hurt themselves. While many have claimed psychedelics saved them from suicide, there's also the risk that the experience could amplify suicidal thoughts and ideation, so appropriate aftercare will be needed for these individuals.

EPILEPSY AND HISTORY OF SEIZURES

Although not explicitly disqualified from all clinical trials with psychedelics, there is some concern for those with epilepsy or a history of seizures taking psilocybin. Giordano tells me the concern isn't for the trip itself, but for the comedown. That's because psilocybin can change the neural chemical balance of someone with epilepsy and can reset their seizure threshold. This risk is increased for those on anti-epilepsy medications, because according to Giordano, "the interaction of the medication with the psilocybin and changing the brain's network activities may be detrimental." I ask him: What if someone has only had one past seizure, should they still avoid psilocybin? He replies that if it was years ago, with no subsequent seizure activity and that person wasn't taking seizure medication, then maybe a mushroom trip could be a possibility. But he also warns that if that person had a substance-induced seizure, then they should avoid psychedelics because there is a risk of "substance induction," which is a type of substance-induced psychosis. Giordano ends our conversation about epilepsy pointing out that there's a caveat, that perhaps people with epilepsy or a

---

135   Lyons, T., et al., "Increased Nature Relatedness and Decreased Authoritarian."

history of seizures could still use psilocybin, just not without clinician approval.

POSSIBLE DRUG INTERACTIONS

Like I described in Chapter I, psilocybin is a relatively safe compound,[136] especially when used mindfully with adequate preparation. But problems can arise once you start mixing psilocybin with other substances, including prescriptions, supplements, other ceremonial plants, and recreational drugs. The following list of possible drug interactions is just a starting point, highlighting frequently asked-about drug mixes. It's by no means an official reference, especially if you're considering taking psilocybin while on prescription medication. I urge you to continue doing your research and speak with a physician before mixing any types of substances. And when it comes to recreational mixes, remember that psilocybin is very powerful and sacred, and the safest way to use it is on its own, in a secure and prepared environment. "Once you start adding things into the soup, so to speak, the flavor has the potential to change," Giordano says to highlight this fact, "and you simply can't guarantee what that's going to be like."

ANTIDEPRESSANTS: SSRIs AND SNRIs

The main prescription mix that experts warn against is combining psilocybin with antidepressants like SSRIs and

---

136   Nutt, D., et al., "Drug Harms in the UK." (Mushrooms found to be the least harmful drug in the UK.)

serotonin-norepinephrine reuptake inhibitors (SNRIs) (some popular brand names include Prozac, Zoloft, Paxil, Lexapro, Cymbalta, and Effexor). That's because these drugs also affect the serotonin system, the main receptor system that psilocybin interacts with. Giordano explains that these types of antidepressants already make more serotonin available in the space between nerve cells in the brain. And so, when psilocybin also acts on that system, there's a risk of essentially "overdosing" on serotonin, known as "serotonin syndrome." Giordano says symptoms could include sweating, agitation, elevation in body temperature, sleeplessness, cardiac effects, and a "very peculiar motor activity called wet dog shakes."

But when I ask other experts about the risk of serotonin syndrome, they explain it's very rare to occur from combining only psilocybin and antidepressants. Zelfand says she'd be much more worried if someone was mixing multiple drugs. For example, combining psilocybin with an antidepressant and another psychedelic like DMT, an empathogen like MDMA, or the popular supplement 5-HTP, would pose a much higher risk. Zelfand reiterates something I've heard in the community and through my interviews with mushroom users, that people who take psilocybin while on SSRI or SNRI antidepressants simply feel less of the psychedelic effects or have to take more shrooms than their friends to trip at all.

Bottom line? I would definitely approach this mix with caution. It's also important to keep in mind that stopping your antidepressants to take psilocybin comes with its own risks, especially withdrawal, depression, and suicidal ideation. Plus, most antidepressants have a very long half-life, meaning you can't stop taking them just the day of your planned mushroom trip.

To get an SSRI completely out of your system, it's best to wait at least two weeks since your last dose before taking psilocybin. And always consult your doctor when weaning off prescription medication.

BUPROPION (WELLBUTRIN)

The last thing worth mentioning about antidepressants is not all of them affect the brain's serotonin system. For example, bupropion, which is the main ingredient of the popular antidepressant Wellbutrin, works by affecting the brain's dopamine system and so poses less of a risk when mixing with psilocybin, says both Giordano and Zelfand. What's more, Wellbutrin shouldn't dull the effects of your trip like SSRI or SNRI antidepressants likely will.

MOOD STABILIZERS

Through talking to people, I've found that mood stabilizers are another common prescription for those struggling with depression, anxiety, and related mood disorders in the United States. The same precaution goes for most mood stabilizers as antidepressants: mixing them isn't the best idea, but the risk increases if the medication interacts with the serotonin system, or if you mix multiple drugs. I ask doctors about any potential risk of mixing psilocybin with two popular mood stabilizers, Lamictal (lamotrigine) and lithium, and learn something interesting about each.

While both Giordano and Zelfand don't note any significant risk of combing mushrooms with Lamictal, Giordano expresses concern about lithium. First, he explains lithium has a downstream effect on the serotonin system, and so it's one of the drug interactions that could increase your chance of serotonin syndrome. What's more, mixing the two can also change the way they're each metabolized. And because lithium exists in a very narrow therapeutic window, that can lead to negative consequences, including lithium toxicity, which can be dangerous. Giordano also warns of the possibility for a really heavy comedown in which people can become "profoundly depressed." Overall, his suggestion is not to mix psilocybin with lithium, to avoid a potentially problematic reaction.

BENZODIAZEPINES

Benzodiazepines, or "benzos" like Xanax, Klonopin, and Ativan, are generally used to relieve acute anxiety and can also do so during a distressing psychedelic experience, but with a few caveats. First of all, medications should only be administered by a clinician, so I can't recommend you take one or offer one to another person to relieve a bad trip. That being said, it is pretty common knowledge within the psychedelic community that benzos can help people calm down from really scary and stress-inducing journeys. Zelfand confirms this for me, explaining they can act as a kind of "rip cord" from psychedelic experiences. You'll still be tripping, she says, but you won't be as distressed by it because of the calming effect of the benzodiazepine.

CANNABIS

Mixing psilocybin and cannabis is probably the most popular drug combination. Physiologically, it's pretty safe, unless you have an underlying heart condition, then there's a chance it could be dangerous. But psychologically, the subjective experience of mixing the two substances can be very strong. For me personally, smoking high-THC cannabis while I'm already under the influence of mushrooms really accentuates the psilocybin and can make the psychedelic effects feel much stronger. Especially toward the end of a psilocybin trip when the psychedelic effects are beginning to wear off, smoking a little cannabis can bring me right back to full-on tripping. But I'm a regular cannabis consumer who is comfortable with the mushroom experience, so it's not overwhelming.

If you're inexperienced with both substances, I would say hold off on combining the two, because it can be pretty intense. Especially if you're the type of person for whom using high-THC cannabis makes you anxious, that anxiety-inducing effect will likely be strengthened while also under the influence of psilocybin. Giordano confirms this, explaining that it all comes back to context. If cannabis makes you anxious generally, using it while tripping can change your whole mood state or set to one of anxiety, which can then flavor your trip for the worst.

ALCOHOL

None of the experts I spoke with expressed much concern over mixing alcohol with magic mushrooms, especially in low doses (one or two drinks). I can say from experience that you probably won't crave much alcohol while you're actively tripping because the thought of consuming much of anything is often pretty secondary. Some have said that a drink before a psychedelic experience helps them unwind, but I would also caution it could probably increase your chance of nausea and vomiting. I also wouldn't recommend accepting any mushrooms while you're already in a social drinking situation. It's a common first-trip mistake to take them casually (and drunkenly) in a party setting without any preparation or care taken as to set and setting, which can end in folks having a really overwhelming experience. I personally like a single cold beer after a psychedelic experience, but I like a cold beer after work in general, and often tripping is tiring in a similar way. Plus, it can help me unwind and fall asleep, which can be hard after tripping for several hours.

MDMA

Taking MDMA or Ecstasy with psilocybin (or LSD, for that matter) is a popular recreational mix known as "hippie flipping." But even though people do it and there's a fun nickname for it, it doesn't mean it's completely safe. Giordano expresses a lot of concern when I ask him about this mix. "That combination can cause a rather dramatic depletion of serotonin and the crash effect can be profound," he says. What's more, the risk is increased if you take multiple doses of MDMA throughout the night, then you run the risk of a clinical comedown known as "serotonin rebound syndrome." "Although it's a popular mix because of the way it makes individuals feel acutely, you're really juggling chainsaws with that one," Giordano warns.

DMT, "BOOSTER DOSES," AND OTHER PSYCHEDELICS

Sometimes I hear of people mixing psychedelics. It's commonly either taking a hit of smokable DMT while they're already on psilocybin, or taking a "booster dose" of the same substance a few hours into the experience. While booster doses of psilocybin are basically safe, they're usually not necessary. My biggest concern is that people don't wait long enough for the first dose to fully kick in and end up taking more mushrooms than they're prepared for. If you're set on making a booster dose available,

I would say wait a full 90 minutes to two hours to evaluate how you feel before adding any more medicine into your system.

As far as combining psychedelics, Giordano does not recommend it. Although he admits that mixing LSD and psilocybin would be safer than combining mushrooms with DMT, especially ayahuasca, but also smokable forms of DMT. That's because DMT not only stimulates an increase in the release of serotonin, but it also stimulates tryptamine, which then also binds to serotonin. "You're getting the big whammy there," Giordano warns, and so it's probably best for your brain and your comedown to avoid the mix and experience each substance individually.

GHB AND KETAMINE

The last popular rec mixes I'll highlight are GHB (gamma hydroxybutyrate) and ketamine. GHB is a central nervous system depressant that in high doses or mixed with other downers, like alcohol, causes people to pass out and can blur their memory, making it, unfortunately, an ideal date-rape drug. However, at low doses without alcohol, it has psychoactive effects, like euphoria, and has become popular for clubbing. Mixed with psilocybin or LSD, people report feeling more euphoric, or "floaty, and fluffy."[137] However, it's very dose dependent, and the chance of dosing too much and passing out is high. If you do pass out, then there's a chance of aspirating vomit, which could be lethal, says Giordano. He also warns that people could black out but stay awake, and in the tripping state could do something dangerous or stupid. And of course, if you're using mushrooms for introspection and personal growth, GHB is likely to make

---

137 GHB and LSD. www.bluelight.org/xf/threads/ghb-and-lsd.583551/

your trip harder to recall and so harder to learn from and integrate.

People also combine psilocybin with ketamine, a dissociative anesthetic with psychedelic effects. The effect of this combo is also very dependent on dose because that's how ketamine's psychoactive effects work. At low doses under 50 to 100 mg (depending on body weight), people use ketamine for its euphoric, almost alcohol- or MDMA-like effects, and it's popular at clubs and raves. But at higher doses, anywhere between 100 to 250 mg and above, ketamine produces a strong psychedelic effect, commonly referred to as a "K-hole." And so when combing psilocybin with ketamine, the dose of ketamine will be the biggest predictor of experience. Basically, it can take the psychedelic experience to another level, with much more intense visuals and ego loss for about an hour. But ketamine trips can be harder to navigate, and it's not uncommon to have a negative experience. Ketamine at higher doses can also create a feeling of not being able to move your arms or legs, which can be disconcerting and potentially dangerous. "The experience of the trip is going to be overwhelming and completely encompassing," says Giordano. "There's going to be a loss of external sensation and external control and for many people that is not pleasant." Giordano also warns that dosing ketamine can be tricky, and achieving the desired low-dose effect depends on a lot of factors, like other substances in your system, stress level, and weight. Plus, when the ketamine wears off, it can create intense nausea for some people, which could be exacerbated by the mushrooms, and that can also increase your risk of choking on vomit.

HALLUCINOGEN PERSISTING PERCEPTION DISORDER (HPPD)

When I ask Giordano about these popular drug combinations, he informs me that another risk factor involved in mixing psilocybin with other substances is the possibility of developing hallucinogen persisting perception disorder (HPPD), a condition characterized by lasting visual distortions and sometimes depression and depersonalization. I stop him—isn't there some controversy as to whether HPPD exists at all? In the weeks following our conversation, I do some more research and learn that while the rumor of "permatripping"—where your psychedelic experience never ends and you go insane—seems to be an urban legend, HPPD is real and affects an estimated 4 percent of psychedelic users.[138]

I call Giordano back a month later to talk about it, and he agrees, permatripping isn't real but the symptoms of HPPD are a spectrum, ranging from psychedelic flashbacks to slight visual distortions, like seeing trails, halos, or things in the corner of your eye. Many with HPPD also experience depression and anxiety due to distressing symptoms and some have dissociative episodes known as depersonalization/derealization.[139]

HPPD can go away in time, and folks have found symptom relief from acceptance and mindfulness techniques, as well as doctor-prescribed, antianxiety medications like benzodiazepines and

---

138 Baggott, et al., "Abnormal Visual Experiences in Individuals."

139 Janikian, "The HPPD Debate: Is Hallucinogen Persisting Perception Disorder Real?"

mood stabilizers like Lamictal.[140] However, many people find cannabis can worsen symptoms, as can a night of heavy drinking or other substance use, and Giordano confirms this for me. He also says that regular cannabis consumers are at a higher risk for developing HPPD, as are those who use psychedelics frequently, especially in higher doses, and folks who mix multiple substances. There are also some other risk factors like a possible genetic predisposition of some people, especially those with other underlying mental health and neurological conditions, as well as certain stimuli during the psychedelic experience, like going from extreme dark to light or vice versa, Giordano says.

Many articles online claim LSD is more likely to cause HPPD than psilocybin, but Giordano and another doctor I speak to say it's more likely that people are using LSD more frequently than psilocybin rather than acid being more dangerous than mushrooms. To my knowledge, there haven't been any reported cases of HPPD in recent clinical participants, but because so much care is put into participant selection, set, setting, and preparation, plus the absence of mixing substances, it's not surprising. In general, it's another reason to respect psilocybin's power and take it cleanly in a safe, calm environment.

HEALTHY FREQUENCY OF USE: HOW OFTEN IS TOO OFTEN TO TRIP?

Can you use mushrooms too much? Even though psilocybin-containing mushrooms don't promote "compulsive use" and so

---

140   Hermle, L., et al., "Hallucinogen-Persisting Perception Disorder."

aren't considered addictive like cocaine or opiates, what would constitute overuse? Obviously using more than a microdose every day would be too much, but what about once a week? What about once a month?

The community's general rule of thumb concerning frequency is: "the more profound the experience, the longer you should wait before doing it again," and after a very meaningful trip, you'll likely find yourself needing time to digest the experience before jumping back in. The experts say doing full-dose mushroom trips more than every six months or so is too much mostly because they believe you need about six months to integrate.[141] While I think it's good advice, I also think if you enjoy mushrooms and benefit from them, then they could be used a bit more frequently than twice a year.

To get an idea of what the community thinks, I asked my social media following, and I received an interesting mix of responses. First off, most people told me that yes, you can do mushrooms too often, although a good chunk of people disagreed. Yet, defining "too often" was a little more hazy. Everyone seemed to agree doing mushrooms every day was a bad idea, and many said doing it once a week and even once a month can be too much. Most believe that the effects won't be as strong or significant if you use mushrooms more than once a month or so, and they agree with the experts, that you won't have enough time to really learn from and integrate your experiences if you're having them frequently. My advice? Don't take mushrooms more than quarterly or so, when you think you need or could benefit from them, to keep the experience sacred and significant.

---

141   Fadiman, *The Psychedelic Explorer's Guide.*

Although mushrooms are generally safe, they're still incredibly powerful, and people with certain conditions do need to take extra care. But by not taking them in combination with other substances, and only every few months or less with appropriate preparation, you'll have the safest, most meaningful, and possibly transformative journey.

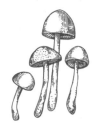

CONCLUSION

Mushrooms are not something to be taken lightly, hence this entire book on how to use them safely. They are powerful substances—even if they're considered harmless physically in moderate doses, they can be emotionally and spiritually intense, both during the trip and in the weeks that follow. But preparation and intentional use are key to having a meaningful experience that isn't needlessly brought down by stress and anxiety.

For your first time consuming mushrooms or any psychedelic (or your first time in years), take it slow. Be gentle with yourself: Start with a low dose in a well-prepared environment to get accustomed to the feeling and to learn what you like and don't in that sensitive state of mind. Read this guide carefully, and keep doing your research by reading other books and resources on the matter, and by talking to people with psychedelic experience.

By treating these sacred fungi with respect and patience, they'll likely show you the same courtesy. Remember, there's no rush or need to get to a heroic dose. This isn't a competition, and the only person you'll end up hurting is yourself. But by taking special care to prepare and integrate, and being mindful of your needs and limits, psilocybin mushrooms might show you a transcendental experience that you can use to transform your life. But the first steps start with you. Be safe out there!

FURTHER READING, VIEWING, AND LISTENING

ONLINE RESOURCES

Beckley Foundation

beckleyfoundation.org

This British NGO funds research into the clinical potential of psychedelic substances.

Blue Light

bluelight.org

Blue Light is an online forum and community for honest drug-harm-reduction information.

Chacruna Institute for Psychedelic Plant Medicine

chacruna.net

The Chacruna Institute is an inclusive organization that provides information on both scientific and ceremonial uses of sacred and psychedelic plants.

Cosmic Sister

www.zoehelene.com

Cosmic Sister is an environmental feminist educational advocacy group supporting women in the psychedelic movement.

DanceSafe

dancesafe.org

This 501(c)(3) public health organization promotes health and safety within the nightlife and electronic music community.

DoubleBlind Magazine

doubleblindmag.com

A biannual print magazine and media company that covers timely, untold stories about the expansion of psychedelics around the globe.

Drug Combination Chart

tripsit.me/tripsit-releases-v3-0-of-its-drug-combination-chart

TripSit offers this very useful online guide on the effects and cautions of combining drugs.

Erowid

erowid.org

A member-supported organization that provides access to reliable, nonjudgmental information about psychoactive plants, chemicals, and related issues.

Flight Instructions

trippingly.net/lsd-studies/2018/5/16/trip-instructions

Bill Richards's instructions for guides and sitters who lead psychedelic sessions.

Heffter Research Institute

heffter.org

The Heffter Research Institute is a 501(c)(3) nonprofit scientific organization that funds psilocybin-assisted therapy trials at prominent research institutions.

Midwest Grow Kits

midwestgrowkits.com

In business for 14 years, this is a popular US supplier of automated mushroom cultivation kits.

Multidisciplinary Association for Psychedelic Studies (MAPS)

maps.org

MAPS is a 501(c)(3) nonprofit research and educational organization that develops medical, legal, and cultural contexts for people to benefit from careful uses of psychedelics and marijuana.

Psychedelic Integration Therapist Database

psychedelic.support

The Psychedelic Support Network lists licensed clinicians who provide psychedelic integration sessions for clients.

Psychedelics Today

psychedelicstoday.com

This media company provides articles, podcasts, workbooks, classes, and other resources about psychedelics.

Shroomery

shroomery.org

An online community that offers accurate information about mushrooms, including effects of shrooms and how to grow magic mushrooms.

Spore Works

sporeworks.com

Spore Works is a legal supplier of "rare and exotic" mushroom spores, including psilocybin-containing species, which you can order from their website.

TripSafe

tripsafe.org

TripSafe is an educational website that provides information on psychedelics including mushrooms, LSD, and others.

Usona Institute

usonainstitute.org

This 501(c)(3) nonprofit medical research organization funds clinical trials on the therapeutic use of psilocybin.

The Women's Visionary Congress
20 Safety Tips for Participating in Ceremonies That Use Psychoactive Substances. https://www.visionarycongress.org/safety-tips-for-participating-in-psychedelic-ceremonies.
The Women's Visionary Congress created this safety checklist for evaluating a potential psychedelic retreat or guided experience.

Zendo Project
zendoproject.org
A MAPS-sponsored peer-support program that trains and provides harm-reduction and trip-sitting services at music festivals.

BOOKS

Acid Test: LSD, Ecstasy, and the Power to Heal by Tom Shroder

The Doors of Perception and Heaven and Hell by Aldous Huxley

DMT: The Spirit Molecule: A Doctor's Revolutionary Research into the Biology of Near-Death and Mystical Experiences by Rick Strassman, MD

How to Change Your Mind: What the New Science of Psychedelics Teaches Us About Consciousness, Dying, Addiction, Depression, and Transcendence by Michael Pollan

Integration Workbook: Planting Seeds for Growth and Change by Psychedelics Today, Kyle Buller, and Joe Moore

LSD, My Problem Child by Albert Hofmann, PhD

Plants of the Gods: Their Sacred, Healing, and Hallucinogenic Powers by Richard Evan Schultes, Albert Hofmann, and Christian Rätsch

The Psilocybin Mushroom Bible: The Definitive Guide to Growing and Using Magic Mushrooms by Virginia Haze and Dr. K Mandrake

Psilocybin Mushrooms of the World: An Identification Guide by Paul Stamets

The Psychedelic Explorer's Guide: Safe, Therapeutic, and Sacred Journeys by James Fadiman, PhD

A Really Good Day: How Microdosing Made a Mega Difference in My Mood, My Marriage, and My Life by Ayelet Waldman

Sacred Knowledge: Psychedelics and Religious Experiences by William Richards

The Wild Kindness: A Psilocybin Odyssey by Bett Williams

VIEWING

Hamilton's Pharmacopeia
vice.com/en_us/topic/hamiltons-pharmacopeia
VICE produces this docuseries on drug effects, origins, and benefits.

Let's Grow Mushrooms! Pf tek
youtu.be/ZHJQrsZFQdE
This is a four-part series of short videos on YouTube that shows how to cultivate mushrooms using the brown rice flour technique (pf tek) and how to make your own DIY grow kit.

Little Saints: Eat a Mushroom, Talk to God
littlesaintsmovie.com
This documentary follows six people who travel to Huautla de Jiménez, Oaxaca, Mexico, to participate in a traditional magic mushroom ceremony.

A New Understanding: The Science of Psilocybin
anewunderstanding.org
This documentary explores the use of psilocybin for end-of-life anxiety, both past and present.

LISTENING

Adventures Through the Mind (podcast) by James W. Jesso
https://www.jameswjesso.com/podcast/

Bill Richards's Playlist for Psilocybin Sessions (music) – Spotify Playlist
open.spotify.com/playlist/4Kvr21ParGx7xI3CqnhXYk?si=apifBFhj
Sz-g8y-Ntpt-6w

Magic Mushrooms Ceremony (music) – Spotify Playlist
open.spotify.com/playlist/6mJ6BQElppq9I2AfWv22IH?si=gJaJI_
TdRAWN5kcMkf7sSw

Music for Mushrooms: A Soundtrack for the Psychedelic Practitioner (music) — East Forest Album
https://music.eastforest.org/album/music-for-mushrooms-a-
soundtrack-for-the-psychedelic-practitioner-2019

Soul Medicine (music) – Spotify Playlist
open.spotify.com/playlist/51v4cno0QBdMIwQuycqutSf?si=
jMF3cAmZTeO229n46ICaoA

BIBLIOGRAPHY

A New Understanding: Science of Psilocybin, directed by Roslyn Dauber, 2015.

Anderson, Thomas, Rotem Petranker, Daniel Rosenbaum, et al. "Microdosing Psychedelics: Personality, Mental Health, and Creativity Differences in Microdosers." *Psychopharmacology (2018). doi:* 10.31234/osf.io/gk4jd.

Baggott, M. J., J. R. Coyle, E. Erowid, et al. "Abnormal Visual Experiences in Individuals with Histories of Hallucinogen Use: A Web-Based Questionnaire." *Drug and Alcohol Dependence 114, no. 1 (2011):* 61–67. doi: 10.1016/j.drugalcdep.2010.09.006.

Beliveau, Vincent, Melanie Ganz, Ling Feng, et al. "A High-Resolution in Vivo Atlas of the Human Brain's Serotonin System." *Journal of Neuroscience 37, no. 1 (2017):* 120–28. doi: 10.1523/JNEUROSCI.2830-16.2016.

Bhagwagar Zubin, Rainer Hinz, Matthew Taylor, et al. "Increased 5-HT(2A) Receptor Binding in Euthymic, Medication-Free Patients Recovered from Depression: A Positron Emission Study with [(11) C]MDL 100,907." *American Journal of Psychiatry 163, no. 9 (2006). doi:* 10.1176/ajp.2006.163.9.1580.

Bluelight.org. "GHB and LSD." Accessed August 26, 2019. www.bluelight.org/xf/threads/ghb-and-lsd.583551.

Boulougouris, Vasileios, Jeffrey Glennon, Trevor Robbins, et al. "Dissociable Effects of Selective 5-HT2A and 5-HT2C Receptor Antagonists on Serial Spatial Reversal Learning in Rats." *Neuropsychopharmacology 33, no. 8 (2008). doi:* 10.1038/sj.npp.1301584.

Buckner, Randy L., J. R. Andrews-Hanna, D. L. Schacter, et al. "The Brain's Default Network." *Annals of the New York Academy of Sciences* 1124, no.1 (2008). doi: 10.1196.annals.1440.011.

Carhart-Harris, Robin L., M. Bolstridge, J. Rucker, et al. "Psilocybin with Psychological Support for Treatment-Resistant Depression." *The Lancet* 3, no. 7 (July 2016): 619-27.

Carhart-Harris, Robin L., Leor Roseman, Mark Bolstridge, et al. "Psilocybin for Treatment-Resistant Depression: fMRI-Measured Brain Mechanisms." *Scientific Reports* 7, no. 1 (2017): 3187. doi: 10.1038/s41598-017-13282-7.

Carhart-Harris, Robin L. and K. J. Friston. "REBUS and the Anarchic Brain: Toward a Unified Model of the Brain Action of Psychedelics." *Pharmacological Reviews* 71, no. 3 (2019): 316-44. doi: 10.1124/pr.118.017160.

Carhart-Harris, Robin, David Erritzoe, Tim Williams, et al. "Neural Correlates of the Psychedelic State as Determined by fMRI Studies with Psilocybin." *Proceedings of the National Academy of Sciences of the United States of America* 109, no. 6 (2012): 2138–43. doi: 10.1073/pnas.1119598109.

Carhart-Harris, Robin L., David Erritzoe, Eline Haijen, et al. "Psychedelics and Connectedness." *Journal of Psychopharmacology* 235, no.2 (2018): 547-50. doi: 10.1007/s00213-107-4701-y.

Carhart-Harris, Robin L. and Guy M. Goodwin. "The Therapeutic Potential of Psychedelic Drugs: Past, Present, and Future." *Neuropsychopharmacology* 42, no. 11 (2017): 2105–13.

Carhart-Harris, Robin L., Robert Leech, Peter Hellyer, et al. "The Entropic Brain: A Theory of Conscious States Informed by Neuroimaging Research with Psychedelic Drugs. *Frontiers in Human Neuroscience* (2014). doi: 10.3389/fnhum.2014.00020.

Carod-Artal, Francisco Javier. "Hallucinogenic Drugs in Pre-Columbian Mesoamerican Cultures." *Neurología* (English Edition) 30, no. 1 (2015): 42–49. doi: 10.1016/j.nrl.2011.07.003.

Clarke, Walter Houston and G. Ray Funkhouser. "Physicians and Researchers Disagree on Psychedelic Drugs." *Psychology Today* 3, no. 11 (1970): 48–50, 70–73.

Costa, P. T., Jr. and R. R. McCrae. "Revised NEO Personality Inventory (NEO-PI-R) and NEO Five Factor Inventory (NEO-FFI)." In *The SAGE Handbook of Personality Theory and Assessment, Vol. 2; Personality Measurement and Testing,* edited by G. J. Boyle, G. Matthews, and D. H. Saklofske, 179–98. Thousand Oaks, CA, US: Sage Publications, Inc., 2008.

Costandi, Mo. "A Brief History of Psychedelic Psychiatry," *The Guardian.* Last modified September 2, 2014, https://www.theguardian.com/science/neurophilosophy/2014/sep/02/psychedelic-psychiatry.

Davey, Christopher G. and Ben J. Harrison. "The Brain's Center of Gravity: How the Default Mode Network Helps Us to Understand the Self." *World Psychiatry* 17, no. 3 (2018): 278–79. doi: 10.10002/wps.20553.

Doblin, Rick. "Pahnke's 'Good Friday Experiment': A Long-Term Follow-Up and Methodological Critique." *The Journal of Transpersonal Psychology* 23, no. 1 (1991): 1-28.

Drug Policy Alliance. "Are Psilocybin Mushrooms Addictive?" Accessed August 26, 2019. www.drugpolicy.org/drug-facts/are-psilocybin-mushrooms-addictive.

Erowid.org. Accessed August 26, 2019.

Erowid. "Psilocybin Mushrooms: Fatalities/Deaths." Accessed August 26, 2019. https://erowid.org/plants/mushrooms/mushrooms_death.shtml.

Fadiman, James and Krob, Sophia. "Microdosing Psychedelics." In *Advances in Psychedelic Medicine*, edited by M. Winkelman and B. Sessa. Santa Barbara, CA: Praeger, 2019.

Fadiman, James. *The Psychedelic Explorer's Guide: Safe, Therapeutic, and Sacred Journeys*. Rochester, Vermont: Park Street Press, 2011.

Farah, Troy. "Inside the Push to Legalize Mushrooms for Depression and PTSD." *Wired*. Last modified February 2, 2019. https://www.wired.com/story/inside-the-push-to-legalize-magic-mushrooms-for-depression-and-ptsd.

Farb, N. A., A. K. Anderson, R. T. Bloch, and Z. V. Segal. "Mood-Linked Responses in Medial Prefrontal Cortex Predict Relapse in Patients With Recurrent Unipolar Depression." *Biological Psychiatry* 70, no.4 (2011): 366–72. doi: 10.1016/j.biopsych.2011.03.009.

Fingelkurts A. A., S. Bagnato, Cristina Boccagni, et al. "DMN Operational Synchrony Relates to Self-Consciousness: Evidence from Patients in Vegetative and Minimally Conscious States." *Open Neuroimaging Journal 6 (2012): 55–68*. doi: 10.2174/1874440001206010055.

Frazer, Jennifer. "Magic Mushroom Drug Evolved to Mess with Insect Brains." October 17, 2018. *Scientific American*. https://blogs.scientificamerican.com/artful-amoeba/magic-mushroom-drug-evolved-to-mess-with-insect-brains.

Garcia-Romeu, A., Alan David, Fire Erowid, et al. "Cessation and Reduction in Alcohol Consumption and Misuse after Psychedelic Use." *Journal of Psychopharmacology* 33, no. 9 (2019). doi: 10.1177/0269881119845793.

Garcia-Romeu, A., R. R. Griffiths, and M. W. Johnson. "Psilocybin-Occasioned Mystical Experiences in the Treatment of Tobacco Addiction." *Current Drug Abuse Reviews 7, no.3 (2014): 157–64.*

Global Drug Survey. Accessed August 26, 2019. www.globaldrug survey.com.

Goldhill, Olivia. *"A Millionaire Couple Is Threatening to Create a Magic Mushroom Monopoly." Quartz.* November 8, 2018. https://qz.com/1454785/a-millionaire-couple-is-threatening-to-create-a-magic-mushroom-monopoly/

Griffiths, Ronald R., Matthew W. Johnson, and William A. Richards. "Psilocybin-Occasioned Mystical-Type Experience in Combination with Meditation and Other Spiritual Practices Produces Enduring Positive Changes in Psychological Functioning in Trait Measures of Prosocial Attitudes and Behaviors." *Journal of Psychopharmacology* 32, no.1, (2018): 49–69. doi: 10.1177/0269881117731279.

Griffiths, Ronald R., William A. Richards, Una D. McCann, et al. "Psilocybin Can Occasion Mystical-Type Experiences Having Substantial and Sustained Personal Meaning and Spiritual Significance." *Journal of Psychopharmacology* 187, no. 3 (2006): 268-83. doi: 10.1007/s00213-006-0457-5.

Griffiths, Ronald R. Matthew Johnson, Michael Carducci, et al. "Psilocybin Produces Substantial and Sustained Decreases in Depression and Anxiety in Patients with Life-Threatening Cancer: A Randomized Double-Blind Trial." *Journal of Psychopharmacology* 30, no. 12. (2016): 1181–97. doi: 10.1177/0269881116675513.

Grob, Charles S., Alicia Danforth, Gurpreet Chopra, et al. "Pilot Study of Psilocybin Treatment for Anxiety in Patients with Advanced-Stage Cancer." *Archives of General Psychiatry* 68, no. 1 (2011): 71-78. doi: 10.1001/archgenpsychiatry.2010.116.

Grof, Stanislav. *LSD Psychotherapy (The Healing Potential of Psychedelic Medicine).* Sarasota, FL: MAPS, 1980.

Heffter Research Institute. "Future Research." Accessed August 26, 2019. https://heffter.org/future-research.

Hendricks, Peter S., Christopher Thorne, Brendan Clark, et al. "Classic Psychedelic Use Is Associated with Reduced Psychological Distress and Suicidality in the United States Adult Population." *Journal of Psychopharmacology* 29, no. 3 (2015): 280–88. doi: 10.1177/0269881114565653.

Hermle, Leo., Melanie Simon, Martin Ruchsow, et al. "Hallucinogen-Persisting Perception Disorder." *Therapeutic Advances in Psychopharmacology* 2, no. 5 (2012) 199–205. doi: 10.1177/2045125312451270.

Hill, Scott. *Confrontation with the Unconscious: Jungian Depth Psychology and Psychedelic Experience.* London: Muswell Hill Press, 2013.

Hofmann, Albert. *LSD, My Problem Child.* Oxford: Oxford University Press, 1979.

Janikian, Michelle. "'The HPPD Debate: Is Hallucinogen Persisting Perception Disorder Real?" *Merry Jane.* September 11, 2019. https://merryjane.com/health/the-hppd-debate-is-hallucinogen-persisting-perception-disorder-real.

Jesso, James W. *The True Light of Darkness.* Calgary, Alberta: SoulsLantern Publishing, 2015.

Johansen, Pal-Orjan and Teri Suzanne Krebs. "Psychedelics Not Linked to Mental Health Problems or Suicidal Behavior: A Population Study." *Journal of Psychopharmacology* 29, no. 3 (2015): 270–79. doi/abs/10.1177/0269881114568039.

Johnson, Matthew W., Albert Garcia-Romeu, Patrick Johnson. "An Online Survey of Tobacco Smoking Cessation Associated with Naturalistic Psychedelic Use." *Journal of Psychopharmacology* 31, no. 7 (2017): 841–50. doi: 10.1177/0269881116684335.

Johnson, Matthew W., William A. Richards, and Roland R. Griffiths. "Human Hallucinogen Research: Guidelines for Safety." *Journal of Psychopharmacology* 22, no. 6 (2008): 603–20. doi: 10.1177/0269881108093587.

Johnson, Matthew W., Albert Garcia Romeu, Roland Griffiths, et al. "Long-Term Follow-Up of Psilocybin-Facilitated Smoking Cessation. *American Journal of Drug and Alcohol Abuse* 43, no. 1 (2017): 55–60. doi: 10.3109/00952990.2016.1170135.

Johnson, Matthew W., Peter Hendricks, Frederick Barrett, et al. "Classic Psychedelics: An Integrative Review of Epidemiology, Therapeutics, Mystical Experience, and Brain Network Function." *Pharmacology and Therapeutics* 197 (2019): doi: 10.1016/j.pharmthera .2018.11.010.

Johnson, Matthew W., William A. Richards, and Roland R. Griffiths. "Human Hallucinogen Research: Guidelines for Safety." *Journal of Psychopharmacology* 22, no. 6 (2008):603–20. doi: 10.1177/0269881108093587.

Johnson, M. W., Roland Griffiths, Peter Hendricks, et al. "The Abuse Potential of Medical Psilocybin According to the 8 Factors of the Controlled Substances Act." *Journal of Neuropharmacology*, no. 142 (2018): 143–66. doi: 10.1016/neuropharm.2018.05.012.

Jung, Carl. *The Collected Works of C. G. Jung. Vol 7. Two Essays in Analytical Psychology*. New Jersey: Princeton University Press, 1953.

Kaplan, J. T., S. I. Gimbel, M. Dehghani, et al. "Processing Narratives Concerning Protected Values: A Cross-Cultural Investigation of Neural Correlates." *Cerebral Cortex* 27, no. 2 (2017): 1428–38. doi: 10.1093/cercor/bhv325.

Kirsch, I., B. J. Deacon, T. B. Huedo-Medina, et al. "Initial Severity and Antidepressant Benefits: A Meta-Analysis of Data Submitted to the Food and Drug Administration." *PLoS Medicine* 5, no. 2 (2008). doi: 10.1371/journal.pmed.0050045.

Leary, Timothy. Ralph Metzner, and Richard Alpert. *The Psychedelic Experience: A Manual Based on the Tibetan Book of the Dead*. New York: Citadel, 2000.

Letcher, Andy. *Shroom: A Cultural History of the Magic Mushroom*. New York: Harper Perennial, 2006.

Lim, T. H., P. N. Ruygrok, and C. A. Wasywich. "A Fatal Case of 'Magic Mushroom' Ingestion in a Heart Transplant Recipient. *Internal Medicine Journal* 42, no. 11 (2012): 1268–9. doi: 10.1111/j.1445-5994.2012.02955.

Little Saints: Eat A Mushroom, Talk to God, directed by Oliver Quintanilla, 2014. www.littlesaintsmovie.com.

Luz Eterna Psilocybin Retreats. "Psilocybin Healing in Oaxaca, Mexico." Accessed October 14, 2019. http://luzeternaretreats.com.

Ly, Calvin, Alexandra Grew, Lindsay Cameron, et al. "Psychedelics Promote Structural and Functional Neural Plasticity." *Cell Reports* 23, no. 11 (2018): :3170–82. doi: 10.1016/j.celrep.2018.05.022.

Lyons, Taylor and Robin L. Carhart-Harris. "Increased Nature Relatedness and Decreased Authoritarian Political Views after Psilocybin for Treatment-Resistant Depression." *Journal of Psychopharmacology* 32, no. 7 (2018): 811–19. doi: 10.1177/0269881117748902.

MacLean, Katherine A., Jeannie-Marie S. Leoutsakos, Matthew W. Johnson, et al. "Factor Analysis of the Mystical Experience Questionnaire: A Study of Experiences Occassioned by the Hallucinogen Psilocybin." *Journal for the Scientific Study of Religion* 51, no. 4 (2012): 721–37. doi: 10.1111/j.1468-5906.2012.01685.

MacLean, Katherine A., Matthew W. Johnson, and Roland R. Griffiths. "Mystical Experiences Occasioned by the Hallucinogen Psilocybin Lead to Increases in the Personality Domain of Openness." *Journal of Psychopharmacology* 25, no. 11. (2011): 1453–1461. doi: 10.1177/0269881111420188.

MacLean, Katherine. "Psychedelic Ethics: The Good, the Bad and the Ugly." Psymposia. Series: Psychedelic Sisters in Arms. www.psymposia .com/magazine/psychedelic-ethics-the-good-the-bad-and-the-ugly.

Maclean, Katherine. "Open Wide and Say Awe," June 20, 2016, https://youtu.be/ZljALxpt3iU.

MAPS. "How to Work with Difficult Experiences," March 3, 2009, https://youtu.be/IaBjoARwlOY.

MAPS. "Psychedelic Integration List." Accessed August 26, 2019. https://integration.maps.org.

Markman, Peter and Roberta Markman. *Masks of the Spirit: Image and Metaphor in Mesoamerica.* Berkeley, CA: University of California Press, 1990.

Meyer J. H., Shelley McMain, Sidney Kennedy, et al. "Dysfunctional Attitudes and 5-HT2 Receptors During Depression and Self-Harm." *American Journal of Psychiatry* 160, no. 1 (2003): 90–99. doi: 10.1176/ appi.ajp.160.1.90.

Microdosing Psychedelics. "Drugs and Supplements." Accessed August 26, 2019. https://sites.google.com/view/ microdosingpsychedelics/drugs-and-supplements.

Microdosing Psychedelics. "FAQ on Microdosing." Accessed August 26, 2019. https://sites.google.com/view/microdosingpsychedelics/ faq-on-microdosing?authuser=0.

Microdosing Psychedelics. "Microdosing Psychedelics." Accessed August 26, 2019. https://sites.google.com/view/microdosing psychedelics/home?authuser=0.

Mindspace. "Psychedelic Psychotherapy." Accessed August 26, 2019. https://www.mindspacewellbeing.com/programs/psychedelics-for-clinicians-101-102.

Monroe, Rachel. "Sexual Assault in the Amazon." *The Cut.* January 18, 2017. www.thecut.com/2017/01/sexual-assault-ayahuasca-tourism .html

Moreno, Francisco, Christopher B. Wiegand, Keolani Taitano, et al. "Safety, Tolerability, and Efficacy of Psilocybin in 9 Patients With Obsessive-Compulsive Disorder." *Journal of Clinical Psychiatry* 67, no. 11 (2006): 1735–40.

Multidisciplinary Association for Psychedelic Studies (MAPS). *The Manual of Psychedelic Support.* 2014. Accessed August 26, 2019. https:// psychsitter.com.

Nutt, David J., Leslie King, and Lawrence Phillips. "Drug Harms in the UK: A Multicriteria Decision Analysis." *Lancet* no. 376 (2010): 1558–65. doi: 10.1016/S0140-6736(10)61462-6.

O'Hare, Ryan. "Magic Mushrooms May 'Reset' the Brains of Depressed Patients." October 13, 2017. www.imperial.ac.uk/ news/182410/magic-mushrooms-reset-brains-depressed-patients.

OMNI magazine. Terence McKenna Interview. May 1993. https:// jacobsm.com/deoxy/deoxy.org/t_omni.htm.

Pahnke, Walter Norman. *Drugs and Mysticism: An Analysis of the Relationship between Psychedelic Drugs and Mystical Consciousness.* Boston: Harvard University, 1963.

Passie, Torsten. *The Science of Microdosing Psychedelics.* London: Psychedelic Press, 2019.

Pisano, Vincent D., Nathaniel Putnam, Hannah Kramer, et al. "The Association of Psychedelic Use and Opioid Use Disorders among Illicit Users in the United States." *Journal of Psychopharmacology* 31, no. 5 (2017): 606–13. doi: 10.1177/0269881117691453.

Polito, Vince and Richard J. Stevenson. "A Systematic Study of Microdosing Psychedelics." *PLoS ONE* 14, no. 2 (2019). doi: 10.1371/journal.pone.0211023.

Pollan, Michael. *How to Change Your Mind: What the New Science of Psychedelics Teaches Us about Consciousness, Dying, Addiction, Depression, and Transcendence.* London: Penguin Press, 2018.

Prochazkova, Luisa, Dominique P. Lippelt, Lorenza Colzato, et al. "Exploring the Effect of Microdosing Psychedelics on Creativity in an Open-Label Natural Setting." *Psychopharmacology* 235, no. 12 (2018): 3401-13. doi: 10.1007/s00213-018-5049-7.

Psychedelic Support. Psychedelic Integration Therapist Database. Accessed August 26, 2019. https://psychedelic.support/network.

Psychedelic Times Staff. "Integrating a Psychedelic Experience through Personal and Spiritual Practices." *Psychedelic Times.* August 8, 2016. https://psychedelictimes.com/integrating-a-psychedelic-experience-through-personal-and-spiritual-practices.

Reddit Forum. "Negative Experiences: Microdosing." Accessed August 26, 2019 https://www.reddit.com/r/microdosing/comments/80Iy8k/negative_experiences/.

Reynolds, Hannah T., Vinod Vijayakumar, Emile Gluck-Thaler, et al. "Horizontal Gene Cluster Transfer Increased Hallucinogenic Mushroom Diversity." *Evolution Letters* 2, no. 2 (2018): 88-101. doi: 10.1002/evl3.42.

Richards, William A. "Flight Instructions." Trippingly.net. July 10, 2018. www.trippingly.net/lsd-studies/2018/5/16/trip-instructions.

Richards, William A. "Sacred Knowledge: Just Because You're Mortal Is No Reason to Be Depressed," filmed at Breaking Conventions August 8, 2017. www.youtube.com/watch?v=oV3a2G9GS_E.

Richards, William A. *Sacred Knowledge: Psychedelics and Religious Experiences.* New York: Columbia University Press, 2015.

Richards, William A. "Navigation within Consciousness: Insight from Four Decades of Psychotherapy Research with Imagery, Music, and Entheogens." *Journal of the Association for Music and Imagery* 9 (2003–2004). https://procrastinative.ninja/data/William%20Bill%20Richards%20-%20Flight%20Instructions.pdf.

Ross, Stephen, et al. "Rapid and Sustained Symptoms Reduction Following Psilocybin Treatment for Anxiety and Depression in Patients with Life-Threatening Cancer: A Randomized Controlled Trial." *Journal of Psychopharmacology* 30, no. 12 (2016): 1165 80. doi: 10.1177/0269881116675512.

Samorini, Giogrio. "The Oldest Representations of Hallucinogenic Mushrooms in the World." *INTEGRATION,* no. 2 (1992).

Samorini, Giorgio. "The Oldest Archaeological Data Evidencing the Relationship of Homo Sapiens with Psychoactive Plants: A Worldwide Overview." *Journal of Psychedelic Studies.* doi: 10.1556/2054.2019.008.

Schultes, Richard Evans, Albert Hoffman, and Christian Rätsch. *Plants of the Gods: Their Sacred, Healing, and Hallucinogenic Powers.* Rochester: Healing Arts Press, 1998.

Sewell, R. A., J. H. Halpern, and H. G. Pope, Jr. "Response of Cluster Headache to Psilocybin and LSD." *Neurology* 66, no. 12 (2006). doi: 10.1212/01.wnl.0000219761.05466.43.

Shulgin, Ann. "Psychedelic Psychotherapy and the Shadow." Accessed August 26, 2019. http://www.matrixmasters.net/podcasts/TRANSCRIPTS/AnnShulgin-TheShadow1.html.

Smart R. G., T. Storm, E. F. Baker, et al. "A Controlled Study of Lysergide in the Treatment of Alcoholism: The Effects on Drinking Behavior." *Quarterly Journals of Studies on Alcohol* 27, no. 3 (1966): 469–82. https://www.ncbi.nlm.nih.gov/pubmed/5970697/.

Smith, Patrick. "Meet the People Who Microdose Psychedelics to Treat ADHD." *The Third Wave*. August 1, 2017. https://thethirdwave.co/microdosing-adhd/.

Solon, Olivia. "Under Pressure, Silicon Valley Workers Turn to LSD Microdosing." *Wired*. August 24, 2016. www.wired.co.uk/article/lsd-microdosing-drugs-silicon-valley.

Stamets, Paul. *Psilocybin Mushrooms of the World: An Identification Guide.* Berkeley, CA: Ten Speed Press, 1996.

Stamets, Paul and Joe Rogan. "1035: Joe Rogan Experience," November 7, 2017, www.youtube.com/watch?v=mPqWstVnRjQ.

Stolaroff, Myron. "Using Psychedelics Wisely." *GNOSIS Magazine* no. 26, (1993).

Strassman, R. J, and C. R. Qualls. "Dose-Response Study of N,N-dimethyltryptamine in Humans: I. Neuroendocrine, Autonomic, and Cardiovascular Effects." *Archives of General Psychiatry* 51, no. 2 (1994): 85-97.

Strassman, Rick, S. Wojtowicz, L. E. Luna, and E. Frecka. *Inner Paths to Outer Space: Journeys to Alien Worlds through Psychedelics and Other Spiritual Technologies.* Rochester, VT: Park Street Press, 2008.

The Buena Vida homepage. Accessed August 26, 2019. www.thebuena vida.net

Usona Institute. "Major Depressive Disorder and Psilocybin Clinical Trial." Accessed August 26, 2019. https://usonaclinicaltrials.org/major-depressive-disorder-psilocybin-clinical-trial-psil201.

Vollenweider, Franz X., Margreet Vollenweider-Scherpenhuyzen, Andreas Bäbler, et al. "Psilocybin Induces Schizophrenia-Like Psychosis in Humans via a Serotonin-2 Agonist Action." *NeuroReport* 9, no. 17 (1998): 3897–3902.

Waldman, Ayelet. *A Really Good Day: How Microdosing Made a Mega Difference in my Mood, My Marriage, and My Life.* New York: Knopf, 2017.

Watts, Rosalind and J. Luoma. (2019, in press). "The Use of the Psychological Flexibility Model to Support Psychedelic Assisted Therapy."

Watts, Rosalind, Camilla Day, Jacob Krzanowski, et al. "Patients' Accounts of Increased 'Connectedness' and 'Acceptance' after Psilocybin for Treatment-Resistant Depression." *Journal of Humanistic Psychology* 57 no. 5 (2017): 1–45. doi: 10.1177/0022167817709585.

Wikipedia. "List of Psilocybin Mushroom Species." Accessed August 26, 2019. https://en.wikipedia.org/w/index.php?title=List_of_psilocybin_mushroom_species&oldid=909787559.

Women's Visionary Congress. "20 Safety Tips for Those Participating in Ceremonies That Use Psychoactive Substances." Accessed September 23, 2019. https://www.visionarycongress.org/safety-tips-for-participating-in-psychedelic-ceremonies.

Woods, Baynard. "Baltimore Psychologist Pioneers Team Using Psychedelics As 'Sacred Medicine.'" *The Guardian.* January 10, 2016. https://www.theguardian.com/us-news/2016/jan/10/baltimore-psychologist-pioneers-team-using-psychedelics-as-sacred-medicine.

World Health Organization. "Depression." Last modified March 22, 2018. https://www.who.int/news-room/fact-sheets/detail/depression.

Yanakieva, Steliana, et al. "The Effects of Microdose LSD on Time Perception: A Randomized, Double-Blind, Placebo-Controlled Trial." *Psychopharmacology* 236, no. 4 (2019): 1159–70.

Yensen, Richard and Donna A. Dryer. "Thirty Years of Psychedelic Research: The Spring Grove Experiment and Its Sequels." (1992). https://www.researchgate.net/publication/309477954_Thirty_Years_of_Psychedelic_Research_The_Spring_Grove_Experiment_and_Its_Sequels.

INDEX

ACKNOWLEDGMENTS

First, I'd like to thank my partner, Martin Clarke, for supporting me (and keeping me fed) through writing this book and being my person through thick and thin. To my family, especially my parents, Kathleen and Joe, and my brother, Nick, for being proud of my work no matter what obscure corner of culture it takes me to.

Many thanks to Jessica Grotfeldt and Amanda Schendel for inviting me to join their magical mushroom retreat, and to all the people who shared that experience with me and taught me so much. To all the mushroom people and microdosers who shared their intimate details with me, including Ashley Manta, Tyler Hurst, Rachelle Lynn Gordon, Leland Radovanovic, Sarah ElSayed, Lindsay Krause, Roberto Rivera, William Sumner, and all those who wish to remain anonymous.

Super big thanks to all the experts who took time out of their busy lives to answer my questions, especially Bill Richards, Elizabeth Nielson, Laura Guzmán Davalos, Peter Hendricks, Ros Watts, Inti García Flores, Erica Zelfand, James Giordano, Joe Moore, and Christopher Casuse.

Huge appreciation to my editor at *Playboy*, Ariela Kozin, for taking a chance on me and encouraging me to explore other substances besides cannabis in my work. Endless gratitude to my old boss at *Herb* and now editor-in-chief at *DoubleBlind Magazine*, Shelby Hartman, for continuing to help shape and improve my writing and reporting (we've still got a long way to go!). Big thanks to Ruth Seeley for recommending me for this project, or I may never have heard of this opportunity.

And of course, I'd like to thank Ulysses Press, especially Casie Vogel and Claire Sielaff, for commissioning a whole book on how to use magic mushrooms "like an adult" and helping me share this information with more people.

ABOUT THE AUTHOR

Michelle Janikian is a journalist focused on drug policy, trends, and education. Coming from the legal cannabis industry, where she's helped to shift the plant's image from "destroyer of youth" to legitimate medicine and acceptable pastime, her interests naturally led her to the healing powers of psychedelics. She writes a column for *Playboy* about psychedelics and cannabis, was a staff writer for the cannabis publication *Herb*, and has also been featured in *Rolling Stone*, *DoubleBlind Magazine*, *High Times*, *Merry Jane*, and *Teen Vogue*.

Fed up with the overprescription of psychiatric drugs in the US and in her own life, she began investigating the medicinal value of outlawed and stigmatized plants and substances, including cannabis, psilocybin, and MDMA. Born in New York City and raised in New Jersey, she's lost too many close friends to depression and the opioid epidemic not to share these stories with the world.

Michelle studied writing and psychology at Sarah Lawrence College before traveling extensively through Latin America and eventually settling down in southern Mexico. Find out more on her website: michellejanikian.com or on Instagram @michelle. janikian and Twitter @m0Oshian.